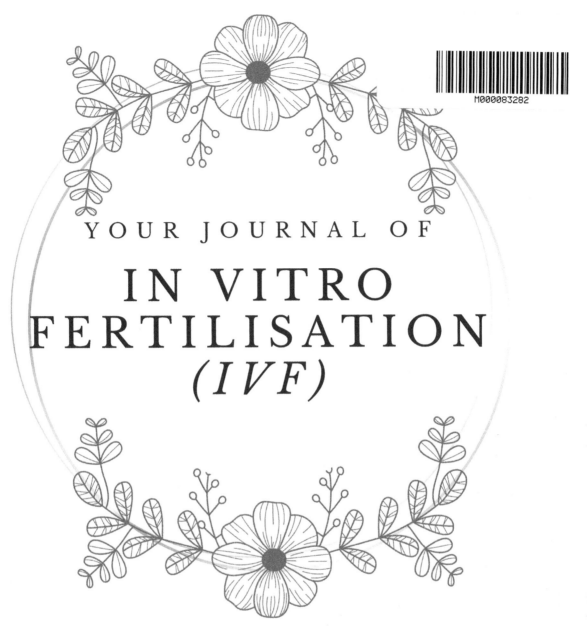

YOUR JOURNAL OF
IN VITRO FERTILISATION
(IVF)

THIS WONT BE EASY - BUT IT WILL BE WORTH IT!

Trying To Conceive (TTC) isn't easy! Use this journal to help you on your journey.
This journal contains....
Everything you need for your TTC journey, you can use if you are trying to conceive naturally but also medically assisted with IVF with medication trackers, fertility trackers, and also(including follicle count & stimulation tracking, medications, doctors appointments, ivf symptoms, transfer days and the two week wait) . And it tracks everything you need! From cervical fluid, mood, temperature, ovulation, medications for those on fertility treatments, and even supplements!

Lined journal pages to write your thoughts, jot down doctors appointments, baby names, and whatever else you want to write about!

Beautiful quotes with illustrations through-out, affirmations and gratitude prompts. TTC can be an emotional roller-coaster! These are in the book to help refocus your thoughts away from negativity and and instead thinking about how precious life is - and why you are on this journey.

Wishing you luck and baby dust.

DAILY ENERGY VS MOOD TRACKER

TRACK YOUR DAILY ENERGY AND MOOD, AS WELL AS DETAILS IN THE NOTES SECTION TO SPOT TRIGGERS.

100						
75						
50						
25						
0	MONDAY	TUESDAY	WEDNESDAY	THURSDAY	FRIDAY	SATURDAY	SUNDAY

FATIGUE/ENERGY

MOOD/ ANXIETYY

FERTILITY TRACKER

CYCLE DAY	1	2	3	4	5	6	7	8	9	10
DATE										
DAY OF THE WEEK										
INTERCOURSE Y/N										
WAKING TEMP.										
CERVICAL FLUID Y/N										
CERVICAL FLUID KEY FOR TYPES	EGGWHITE LIKE SLIPPERY, STRETCHY (E)		CREAMY OPAQUE, MILKY, LOTION-LIKE (C)		STICKY RUBBERY, CRUMBLES, CEMENT (S)		BLEEDING (B)		Use this key to track your cervical fluid changes below.	
CERVICAL FLUID TYPE										
OVULATION Y/N										
OVULATION PAIN Y/N										
LH SPIKE										
STRESS Y/N										
ILLNESS Y/N										
SORE BREASTS Y/N										
CRAMPING										
MOOD TYPE KEY	HORMONAL, MOOD SWINGS, EMOTIONAL (E)		CALM, NEUTRAL, DAY-TO-DAY (C)		ANXIOUS, DEPRESSED, STRESSED. (S)		HAPPY, ENERGETIC. (H)		Use this key to track your mood changes below.	
MOOD										
BLOATING										

MEDICATION & SUPPLEMENT TRACKING & DOSE

CYCLE DAY	1	2	3	4	5	6	7	8	9	10
MEDICATION NAME EXAMPLE	DOSE	N/A								

FERTILITY TRACKER

CYCLE DAY	11	12	13	14	15	16	17	18	19	20
DATE										
DAY OF THE WEEK										
INTERCOURSE Y/N										
WAKING TEMP.										
CERVICAL FLUID Y/N										
CERVICAL FLUID KEY FOR TYPES	EGGWHITE LIKE (E) SLIPPERY, STRETCHY		CREAMY (C) OPAQUE, MILKY, LOTION-LIKE		STICKY (S) RUBBERY, CRUMBLES, CEMENT		BLEEDING (B)		Use this key to track your cervical fluid changes below.	
CERVICAL FLUID TYPE										
OVULATION Y/N										
OVULATION PAIN Y/N										
LH SPIKE										
STRESS Y/N										
ILLNESS Y/N										
SORE BREASTS Y/N										
CRAMPING										
MOOD TYPE KEY	HORMONAL, (E) MOOD SWINGS, EMOTIONAL		CALM, (C) NEUTRAL, DAY-TO-DAY		ANXIOUS, (S) DEPRESSED, STRESSED.		HAPPY, (H) ENERGETIC.		Use this key to track your mood changes below.	
MOOD										
BLOATING										

MEDICATION & SUPPLEMENT TRACKING & DOSE

CYCLE DAY	11	12	13	14	15	16	17	18	19	20
MEDICATION NAME EXAMPLE	DOSE	N/A								

FERTILITY TRACKER

CYCLE DAY	21	22	23	24	25	26	27	28	29	30
DATE										
DAY OF THE WEEK										
INTERCOURSE Y/N										
WAKING TEMP.										
CERVICAL FLUID Y/N										
CERVICAL FLUID KEY FOR TYPES	EGGWHITE LIKE (E) SLIPPERY, STRETCHY		CREAMY OPAQUE, MILKY, LOTION-LIKE (C)		STICKY (S) RUBBERY, CRUMBLES, CEMENT		BLEEDING (B)		Use this key to track your cervical fluid changes below.	
CERVICAL FLUID TYPE										
OVULATION Y/N										
OVULATION PAIN Y/N										
LH SPIKE										
STRESS Y/N										
ILLNESS Y/N										
SORE BREASTS Y/N										
CRAMPING										
MOOD TYPE KEY	HORMONAL, MOOD SWINGS, EMOTIONAL (E)		CALM, NEUTRAL, DAY-TO-DAY (C)		ANXIOUS, DEPRESSED, STRESSED. (S)		HAPPY, ENERGETIC. (H)		Use this key to track your mood changes below.	
MOOD										
BLOATING										

MEDICATION & SUPPLEMENT TRACKING & DOSE

CYCLE DAY	21	22	23	24	25	26	27	28	29	30
MEDICATION NAME EXAMPLE	DOSE	N/A								

FERTILITY TRACKER

CYCLE DAY	31	32	33	34	35	36	37	38	39	40
DATE										
DAY OF THE WEEK										
INTERCOURSE Y/N										
WAKING TEMP.										
CERVICAL FLUID Y/N										
CERVICAL FLUID KEY FOR TYPES	EGGWHITE LIKE SLIPPERY, STRETCHY (E)		CREAMY OPAQUE, MILKY, LOTION-LIKE (C)		STICKY RUBBERY, CRUMBLES, CEMENT (S)		BLEEDING (B)		Use this key to track your cervical fluid changes below.	
CERVICAL FLUID TYPE										
OVULATION Y/N										
OVULATION PAIN Y/N										
LH SPIKE										
STRESS Y/N										
ILLNESS Y/N										
SORE BREASTS Y/N										
CRAMPING										
MOOD TYPE KEY	HORMONAL, MOOD SWINGS, EMOTIONAL (E)		CALM, NEUTRAL, DAY-TO-DAY (C)		ANXIOUS, DEPRESSED, STRESSED. (S)		HAPPY, ENERGETIC. (H)		Use this key to track your mood changes below.	
MOOD										
BLOATING										

MEDICATION & SUPPLEMENT TRACKING & DOSE

CYCLE DAY	31	32	33	34	35	36	37	38	39	40
MEDICATION NAME EXAMPLE	DOSE	N/A								

MEDICATION LOG   WEEK_____ CYCLE _____ DATE _____

CYCLE DAY / MEDICATION	1	2	3	4	5	6	7	8	9	10
MEDICATION NAME EXAMPLE	DOSE TIMESTAMP									

CYCLE DAY / MEDICATION	11	12	13	14	15	16	17	18	19	20

CYCLE DAY	21	22	23	24	25	26	27	28	29	30
MEDICATION										
MEDICATION NAME EXAMPLE	DOSE TIMESTAMP									

CYCLE DAY	31	32	33	34	35	36	37	38	39	40
MEDICATION										

RESULTS, HORMONE AND SYMPTOM LOG   WEEK_____ CYCLE _____ DATE _____

CYCLE DAY / RESULTS & SYMPTOMS	1	2	3	4	5	6	7	8	9	10
DATE										
BASAL TEMP										
LH										
PROGESTERONE										
OESTROGEN										
ENDOTHICKNESS										
FOLLICLES RIGHT # & SIZE										
FOLLICLES LEFT # & SIZE										
FILL IN YOUR OWN										

CYCLE DAY / RESULTS & SYMPTOMS	11	12	13	14	15	16	17	18	19	20
DATE										
BASAL TEMP										
LH										
PROGESTERONE										
OESTROGEN										
ENDOTHICKNESS										
FOLLICLES RIGHT # & SIZE										
FOLLICLES LEFT # & SIZE										
FILL IN YOUR OWN										

RESULTS, HORMONE AND SYMPTOM LOG   WEEK_____ CYCLE _____ DATE _____

CYCLE DAY / RESULTS & SYMPTOMS	21	22	23	24	25	26	27	28	29	30
DATE										
BASAL TEMP										
LH										
PROGESTERONE										
OESTROGEN										
ENDOTHICKNESS										
FOLLICLES RIGHT # & SIZE										
FOLLICLES LEFT # & SIZE										
FILL IN YOUR OWN										

CYCLE DAY / RESULTS & SYMPTOMS	31	32	33	34	35	36	37	38	39	40
DATE										
BASAL TEMP										
LH										
PROGESTERONE										
OESTROGEN										
ENDOTHICKNESS										
FOLLICLES RIGHT # & SIZE										
FOLLICLES LEFT # & SIZE										
FILL IN YOUR OWN										

WRITE YOUR BLOOD, URINE AND OTHER TEST RESULTS

TEST	RESULT	RESULT	RESULT	RESULT

SYMPTOM TRACKER

DATE	TIME	DURATION	DESCRIPTION
DATE	TIME	DURATION	DESCRIPTION

DOCTORS APPOINTMENTS TIME SHEET

DATE	TIME	DOCTOR & LOCATION	REASON & NOTES

EMERGENCY & DOCTORS CONTACTS

DOCTORS APPOINTMENTS TIME SHEET

DATE	TIME	DOCTOR & LOCATION	REASON & NOTES

EMERGENCY & DOCTORS CONTACTS

_____

_____

_____

_____

_____

_____

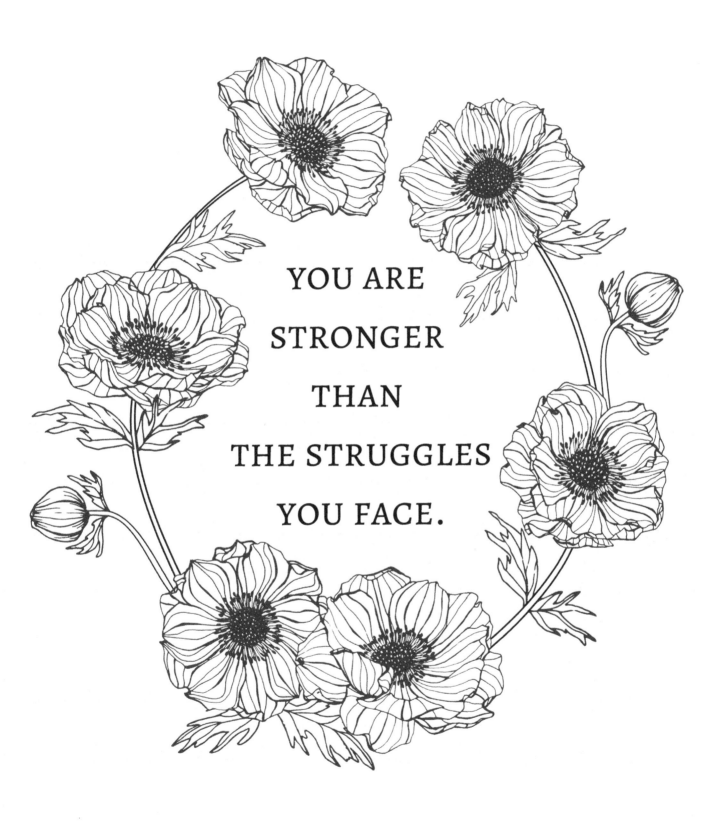

YOU ARE
STRONGER
THAN
THE STRUGGLES
YOU FACE.

WHAT I DID TODAY

MONDAY
_____
_____

TUESDAY
_____
_____

WEDNESDAY
_____
_____

THURSDAY
_____
_____

FRIDAY
_____
_____

SATURDAY
_____
_____

SUNDAY
_____
_____

TODAY I FELT...

MONDAY
_____
_____

TUESDAY
_____
_____

WEDNESDAY
_____
_____

THURSDAY
_____
_____

FRIDAY
_____
_____

SATURDAY
_____
_____

SUNDAY
_____
_____

TWO WEEK WAIT

WHAT I DID TODAY

MONDAY
_____
_____

TUESDAY
_____
_____

WEDNESDAY
_____
_____

THURSDAY
_____
_____

FRIDAY
_____
_____

SATURDAY
_____
_____

SUNDAY
_____
_____

TODAY I FELT...

MONDAY
_____
_____

TUESDAY
_____
_____

WEDNESDAY
_____
_____

THURSDAY
_____
_____

FRIDAY
_____
_____

SATURDAY
_____
_____

SUNDAY
_____
_____

SYMPTOM TRACKER

DATE	TIME	DURATION	DESCRIPTION
DATE	TIME	DURATION	DESCRIPTION

MONTH:

1 2 3 4 5 6 7 8 9 10

11 12 13 14 15 16 17 18 19

20 21 22 23 24 25 26 27 28

29 30 31

MONTH:

1 2 3 4 5 6 7 8 9 10

11 12 13 14 15 16 17 18 19

20 21 22 23 24 25 26 27 28

29 30 31

MONTH:

1 2 3 4 5 6 7 8 9 10

11 12 13 14 15 16 17 18 19

20 21 22 23 24 25 26 27 28

29 30 31

APPOINTMENT, TREATMENT AND PLANNING CALENDAR

CIRCLE GOOD DAYS PUT AN X THROUGH BAD DAYS FOR AN OVERALL VIEW OF IMPROVEMENTS

MONTH:

1	2	3	4	5	6	7
8	9	10	11	12	13	14
15	16	17	18	19	20	21
22	23	24	25	26	27	28
29	30	31				

MONTH:

1	2	3	4	5	6	7
8	9	10	11	12	13	14
15	16	17	18	19	20	21
22	23	24	25	26	27	28
29	30	31				

MONTH:

1	2	3	4	5	6	7
8	9	10	11	12	13	14
15	16	17	18	19	20	21
22	23	24	25	26	27	28
29	30	31				

NOTES:

_____
_____
_____
_____
_____
_____
_____

MONTH:

1	2	3	4	5	6	7
8	9	10	11	12	13	14
15	16	17	18	19	20	21
22	23	24	25	26	27	28
29	30	31				

MONTH:

1	2	3	4	5	6	7
8	9	10	11	12	13	14
15	16	17	18	19	20	21
22	23	24	25	26	27	28
29	30	31				

MONTH:

1	2	3	4	5	6	7
8	9	10	11	12	13	14
15	16	17	18	19	20	21
22	23	24	25	26	27	28
29	30	31				

NOTES:

_____
_____
_____
_____
_____
_____
_____

USE FOR TRANSFER DAYS, THE TWO WEEK WAIT, CYCLE TRACKING, DOCTORS APPOINTMENTS OR JUST "GOOD DAYS" VS "BAD DAYS IN YOUR JOURNEY.

APPOINTMENT, TREATMENT AND PLANNING CALENDAR

CIRCLE GOOD DAYS PUT AN X THROUGH BAD DAYS FOR AN OVERALL VIEW OF IMPROVEMENTS

MONTH:

1	2	3	4	5	6	7
8	9	10	11	12	13	14
15	16	17	18	19	20	21
22	23	24	25	26	27	28
29	30	31				

MONTH:

1	2	3	4	5	6	7
8	9	10	11	12	13	14
15	16	17	18	19	20	21
22	23	24	25	26	27	28
29	30	31				

MONTH:

1	2	3	4	5	6	7
8	9	10	11	12	13	14
15	16	17	18	19	20	21
22	23	24	25	26	27	28
29	30	31				

NOTES:

_____
_____
_____
_____
_____
_____
_____
_____

MONTH:

1	2	3	4	5	6	7
8	9	10	11	12	13	14
15	16	17	18	19	20	21
22	23	24	25	26	27	28
29	30	31				

MONTH:

1	2	3	4	5	6	7
8	9	10	11	12	13	14
15	16	17	18	19	20	21
22	23	24	25	26	27	28
29	30	31				

MONTH:

1	2	3	4	5	6	7
8	9	10	11	12	13	14
15	16	17	18	19	20	21
22	23	24	25	26	27	28
29	30	31				

NOTES:

_____
_____
_____
_____
_____
_____
_____
_____

USE FOR TRANSFER DAYS, THE TWO WEEK WAIT, CYCLE TRACKING, DOCTORS APPOINTMENTS OR JUST "GOOD DAYS" VS "BAD DAYS IN YOUR JOURNEY.

WRITE DOWN ALL THE WAYS IN WHICH YOU ARE STRONG.

ANSWER THESE QUESTIONS TO BREAK OUT OF NEGATIVE THOUGHT PATTERNS AND REFOCUS ON THE THINGS THAT MAKE YOU HAPPY AND GRATEFUL.

DAILY ENERGY VS MOOD TRACKER

TRACK YOUR DAILY ENERGY AND MOOD, AS WELL AS DETAILS IN THE NOTES SECTION TO SPOT TRIGGERS.

100

75

50

25

0 MONDAY   TUESDAY   WEDNESDAY   THURSDAY   FRIDAY   SATURDAY   SUNDAY

FATIGUE/ENERGY   MOOD/ ANXIETYY

FERTILITY TRACKER

CYCLE DAY	1	2	3	4	5	6	7	8	9	10
DATE										
DAY OF THE WEEK										
INTERCOURSE Y/N										
WAKING TEMP.										
CERVICAL FLUID Y/N										
CERVICAL FLUID KEY FOR TYPES	EGGWHITE LIKE, SLIPPERY, STRETCHY (E)		CREAMY OPAQUE, MILKY, LOTION-LIKE (C)		STICKY RUBBERY, CRUMBLES, CEMENT (S)		BLEEDING (B)		Use this key to track your cervical fluid changes below.	
CERVICAL FLUID TYPE										
OVULATION Y/N										
OVULATION PAIN Y/N										
LH SPIKE										
STRESS Y/N										
ILLNESS Y/N										
SORE BREASTS Y/N										
CRAMPING										
MOOD TYPE KEY	HORMONAL, MOOD SWINGS, EMOTIONAL (E)		CALM, NEUTRAL, DAY-TO-DAY (C)		ANXIOUS, DEPRESSED, STRESSED. (S)		HAPPY, ENERGETIC. (H)		Use this key to track your mood changes below.	
MOOD										
BLOATING										

MEDICATION & SUPPLEMENT TRACKING & DOSE

CYCLE DAY	1	2	3	4	5	6	7	8	9	10
MEDICATION NAME EXAMPLE	DOSE	N/A								

FERTILITY TRACKER

CYCLE DAY	11	12	13	14	15	16	17	18	19	20
DATE										
DAY OF THE WEEK										
INTERCOURSE Y/N										
WAKING TEMP.										
CERVICAL FLUID Y/N										
CERVICAL FLUID KEY FOR TYPES	EGGWHITE LIKE (E) SLIPPERY, STRETCHY		CREAMY (C) OPAQUE, MILKY, LOTION-LIKE		STICKY (S) RUBBERY, CRUMBLES, CEMENT		BLEEDING (B)		Use this key to track your cervical fluid changes below.	
CERVICAL FLUID TYPE										
OVULATION Y/N										
OVULATION PAIN Y/N										
LH SPIKE										
STRESS Y/N										
ILLNESS Y/N										
SORE BREASTS Y/N										
CRAMPING										
MOOD TYPE KEY	HORMONAL, (E) MOOD SWINGS, EMOTIONAL		CALM, (C) NEUTRAL, DAY-TO-DAY		ANXIOUS, (S) DEPRESSED, STRESSED.		HAPPY, (H) ENERGETIC.		Use this key to track your mood changes below.	
MOOD										
BLOATING										

MEDICATION & SUPPLEMENT TRACKING & DOSE

CYCLE DAY	11	12	13	14	15	16	17	18	19	20
MEDICATION NAME EXAMPLE	DOSE	N/A								

FERTILITY TRACKER

CYCLE DAY	21	22	23	24	25	26	27	28	29	30
DATE										
DAY OF THE WEEK										
INTERCOURSE Y/N										
WAKING TEMP.										
CERVICAL FLUID Y/N										
CERVICAL FLUID KEY FOR TYPES	EGGWHITE LIKE (E) SLIPPERY, STRETCHY		CREAMY (C) OPAQUE, MILKY, LOTION-LIKE		STICKY (S) RUBBERY, CRUMBLES, CEMENT		BLEEDING (B)		Use this key to track your cervical fluid changes below.	
CERVICAL FLUID TYPE										
OVULATION Y/N										
OVULATION PAIN Y/N										
LH SPIKE										
STRESS Y/N										
ILLNESS Y/N										
SORE BREASTS Y/N										
CRAMPING										
MOOD TYPE KEY	HORMONAL, (E) MOOD SWINGS, EMOTIONAL		CALM, (C) NEUTRAL, DAY-TO-DAY		ANXIOUS, (S) DEPRESSED, STRESSED.		HAPPY, (H) ENERGETIC.		Use this key to track your mood changes below.	
MOOD										
BLOATING										

MEDICATION & SUPPLEMENT TRACKING & DOSE

CYCLE DAY	21	22	23	24	25	26	27	28	29	30
MEDICATION NAME EXAMPLE	DOSE	N/A								

FERTILITY TRACKER

CYCLE DAY	31	32	33	34	35	36	37	38	39	40
DATE										
DAY OF THE WEEK										
INTERCOURSE Y/N										
WAKING TEMP.										
CERVICAL FLUID Y/N										
CERVICAL FLUID KEY FOR TYPES	EGGWHITE LIKE (E) SLIPPERY, STRETCHY		CREAMY (C) OPAQUE, MILKY, LOTION-LIKE		STICKY (S) RUBBERY, CRUMBLES, CEMENT		BLEEDING (B)		Use this key to track your cervical fluid changes below.	
CERVICAL FLUID TYPE										
OVULATION Y/N										
OVULATION PAIN Y/N										
LH SPIKE										
STRESS Y/N										
ILLNESS Y/N										
SORE BREASTS Y/N										
CRAMPING										
MOOD TYPE KEY	HORMONAL, (E) MOOD SWINGS, EMOTIONAL		CALM, (C) NEUTRAL, DAY-TO-DAY		ANXIOUS, (S) DEPRESSED, STRESSED.		HAPPY, (H) ENERGETIC.		Use this key to track your mood changes below.	
MOOD										
BLOATING										

MEDICATION & SUPPLEMENT TRACKING & DOSE

CYCLE DAY	31	32	33	34	35	36	37	38	39	40
MEDICATION NAME EXAMPLE	DOSE	N/A								

MEDICATION LOG　　　WEEK＿＿＿＿＿＿＿　CYCLE ＿＿＿＿＿＿＿　DATE ＿＿＿＿＿＿＿

CYCLE DAY / MEDICATION	1	2	3	4	5	6	7	8	9	10
MEDICATION NAME EXAMPLE	DOSE TIMESTAMP									

CYCLE DAY / MEDICATION	11	12	13	14	15	16	17	18	19	20

MEDICATION LOG   WEEK_____ CYCLE _____ DATE _____

CYCLE DAY / MEDICATION	21	22	23	24	25	26	27	28	29	30
MEDICATION NAME EXAMPLE	DOSE TIMESTAMP									

CYCLE DAY / MEDICATION	31	32	33	34	35	36	37	38	39	40

RESULTS, HORMONE AND SYMPTOM LOG   WEEK_____ CYCLE _____ DATE _____

CYCLE DAY / RESULTS & SYMPTOMS	1	2	3	4	5	6	7	8	9	10
DATE										
BASAL TEMP										
LH										
PROGESTERONE										
OESTROGEN										
ENDOTHICKNESS										
FOLLICLES RIGHT # & SIZE										
FOLLICLES LEFT # & SIZE										
FILL IN YOUR OWN										

CYCLE DAY / RESULTS & SYMPTOMS	11	12	13	14	15	16	17	18	19	20
DATE										
BASAL TEMP										
LH										
PROGESTERONE										
OESTROGEN										
ENDOTHICKNESS										
FOLLICLES RIGHT # & SIZE										
FOLLICLES LEFT # & SIZE										
FILL IN YOUR OWN										

RESULTS, HORMONE AND SYMPTOM LOG   WEEK_____ CYCLE _____ DATE _____

CYCLE DAY RESULTS & SYMPTOMS	21	22	23	24	25	26	27	28	29	30
DATE										
BASAL TEMP										
LH										
PROGESTERONE										
OESTROGEN										
ENDOTHICKNESS										
FOLLICLES RIGHT # & SIZE										
FOLLICLES LEFT # & SIZE										
FILL IN YOUR OWN										

CYCLE DAY RESULTS & SYMPTOMS	31	32	33	34	35	36	37	38	39	40
DATE										
BASAL TEMP										
LH										
PROGESTERONE										
OESTROGEN										
ENDOTHICKNESS										
FOLLICLES RIGHT # & SIZE										
FOLLICLES LEFT # & SIZE										
FILL IN YOUR OWN										

WRITE YOUR BLOOD, URINE AND OTHER TEST RESULTS

TEST	RESULT	RESULT	RESULT	RESULT

MONTH:

1 2 3 4 5 6 7 8 9 10

11 12 13 14 15 16 17 18 19

20 21 22 23 24 25 26 27 28

29 30 31

MONTH:

1 2 3 4 5 6 7 8 9 10

11 12 13 14 15 16 17 18 19

20 21 22 23 24 25 26 27 28

29 30 31

MONTH:

1 2 3 4 5 6 7 8 9 10

11 12 13 14 15 16 17 18 19

20 21 22 23 24 25 26 27 28

29 30 31

APPOINTMENT, TREATMENT AND PLANNING CALENDAR

CIRCLE GOOD DAYS PUT AN X THROUGH BAD DAYS FOR AN OVERALL VIEW OF IMPROVEMENTS

MONTH:

1	2	3	4	5	6	7
8	9	10	11	12	13	14
15	16	17	18	19	20	21
22	23	24	25	26	27	28
29	30	31				

MONTH:

1	2	3	4	5	6	7
8	9	10	11	12	13	14
15	16	17	18	19	20	21
22	23	24	25	26	27	28
29	30	31				

MONTH:

1	2	3	4	5	6	7
8	9	10	11	12	13	14
15	16	17	18	19	20	21
22	23	24	25	26	27	28
29	30	31				

NOTES:

_____

_____

_____

_____

_____

_____

_____

MONTH:

1	2	3	4	5	6	7
8	9	10	11	12	13	14
15	16	17	18	19	20	21
22	23	24	25	26	27	28
29	30	31				

MONTH:

1	2	3	4	5	6	7
8	9	10	11	12	13	14
15	16	17	18	19	20	21
22	23	24	25	26	27	28
29	30	31				

MONTH:

1	2	3	4	5	6	7
8	9	10	11	12	13	14
15	16	17	18	19	20	21
22	23	24	25	26	27	28
29	30	31				

NOTES:

_____

_____

_____

_____

_____

_____

_____

_____

USE FOR TRANSFER DAYS, THE TWO WEEK WAIT, CYCLE TRACKING, DOCTORS APPOINTMENTS OR JUST "GOOD DAYS" VS "BAD DAYS IN YOUR JOURNEY.

APPOINTMENT, TREATMENT AND PLANNING CALENDAR

CIRCLE GOOD DAYS PUT AN X THROUGH BAD DAYS FOR AN OVERALL VIEW OF IMPROVEMENTS

MONTH:

1	2	3	4	5	6	7
8	9	10	11	12	13	14
15	16	17	18	19	20	21
22	23	24	25	26	27	28
29	30	31				

MONTH:

1	2	3	4	5	6	7
8	9	10	11	12	13	14
15	16	17	18	19	20	21
22	23	24	25	26	27	28
29	30	31				

MONTH:

1	2	3	4	5	6	7
8	9	10	11	12	13	14
15	16	17	18	19	20	21
22	23	24	25	26	27	28
29	30	31				

NOTES:

_____
_____
_____
_____
_____
_____
_____
_____

MONTH:

1	2	3	4	5	6	7
8	9	10	11	12	13	14
15	16	17	18	19	20	21
22	23	24	25	26	27	28
29	30	31				

MONTH:

1	2	3	4	5	6	7
8	9	10	11	12	13	14
15	16	17	18	19	20	21
22	23	24	25	26	27	28
29	30	31				

MONTH:

1	2	3	4	5	6	7
8	9	10	11	12	13	14
15	16	17	18	19	20	21
22	23	24	25	26	27	28
29	30	31				

NOTES:

_____
_____
_____
_____
_____
_____
_____
_____

USE FOR TRANSFER DAYS, THE TWO WEEK WAIT, CYCLE TRACKING, DOCTORS APPOINTMENTS OR JUST "GOOD DAYS" VS "BAD DAYS IN YOUR JOURNEY.

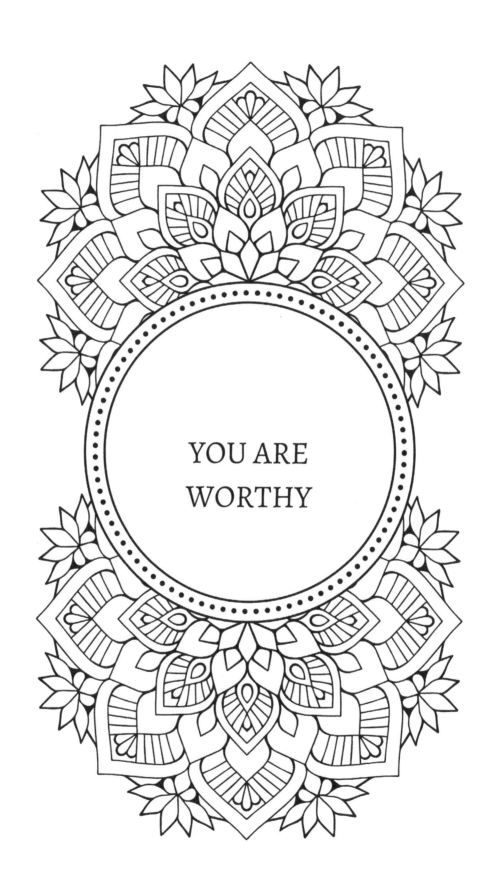

YOU ARE
WORTHY

DAILY ENERGY VS MOOD TRACKER

TRACK YOUR DAILY ENERGY AND MOOD, AS WELL AS DETAILS IN THE NOTES SECTION TO SPOT TRIGGERS.

100

75

50

25

0   MONDAY   TUESDAY   WEDNESDAY   THURSDAY   FRIDAY   SATURDAY   SUNDAY

FATIGUE/ENERGY   MOOD/ ANXIETYY

FERTILITY TRACKER

CYCLE DAY	1	2	3	4	5	6	7	8	9	10
DATE										
DAY OF THE WEEK										
INTERCOURSE Y/N										
WAKING TEMP.										
CERVICAL FLUID Y/N										
CERVICAL FLUID KEY FOR TYPES	EGGWHITE LIKE (E) SLIPPERY, STRETCHY		CREAMY (C) OPAQUE, MILKY, LOTION-LIKE		STICKY (S) RUBBERY, CRUMBLES, CEMENT		BLEEDING (B)		Use this key to track your cervical fluid changes below.	
CERVICAL FLUID TYPE										
OVULATION Y/N										
OVULATION PAIN Y/N										
LH SPIKE										
STRESS Y/N										
ILLNESS Y/N										
SORE BREASTS Y/N										
CRAMPING										
MOOD TYPE KEY	HORMONAL, (E) MOOD SWINGS, EMOTIONAL		CALM, (C) NEUTRAL, DAY-TO-DAY		ANXIOUS, (S) DEPRESSED, STRESSED.		HAPPY, (H) ENERGETIC.		Use this key to track your mood changes below.	
MOOD										
BLOATING										

MEDICATION & SUPPLEMENT TRACKING & DOSE

CYCLE DAY	1	2	3	4	5	6	7	8	9	10
MEDICATION NAME EXAMPLE	DOSE	N/A								

FERTILITY TRACKER

CYCLE DAY	11	12	13	14	15	16	17	18	19	20
DATE										
DAY OF THE WEEK										
INTERCOURSE Y/N										
WAKING TEMP.										
CERVICAL FLUID Y/N										
CERVICAL FLUID KEY FOR TYPES	EGGWHITE LIKE SLIPPERY, STRETCHY (E)		CREAMY OPAQUE, MILKY, LOTION-LIKE (C)		STICKY RUBBERY, CRUMBLES, CEMENT (S)		BLEEDING (B)		Use this key to track your cervical fluid changes below.	
CERVICAL FLUID TYPE										
OVULATION Y/N										
OVULATION PAIN Y/N										
LH SPIKE										
STRESS Y/N										
ILLNESS Y/N										
SORE BREASTS Y/N										
CRAMPING										
MOOD TYPE KEY	HORMONAL, MOOD SWINGS, EMOTIONAL (E)		CALM, NEUTRAL, DAY-TO-DAY (C)		ANXIOUS, DEPRESSED, STRESSED. (S)		HAPPY, ENERGETIC. (H)		Use this key to track your mood changes below.	
MOOD										
BLOATING										

MEDICATION & SUPPLEMENT TRACKING & DOSE

CYCLE DAY	11	12	13	14	15	16	17	18	19	20
MEDICATION NAME EXAMPLE	DOSE	N/A								

FERTILITY TRACKER

CYCLE DAY	21	22	23	24	25	26	27	28	29	30
DATE										
DAY OF THE WEEK										
INTERCOURSE Y/N										
WAKING TEMP.										
CERVICAL FLUID Y/N										
CERVICAL FLUID KEY FOR TYPES	EGGWHITE LIKE SLIPPERY, STRETCHY (E)		CREAMY OPAQUE, MILKY, LOTION-LIKE (C)		STICKY RUBBERY, CRUMBLES, CEMENT (S)		BLEEDING (B)		Use this key to track your cervical fluid changes below.	
CERVICAL FLUID TYPE										
OVULATION Y/N										
OVULATION PAIN Y/N										
LH SPIKE										
STRESS Y/N										
ILLNESS Y/N										
SORE BREASTS Y/N										
CRAMPING										
MOOD TYPE KEY	HORMONAL, MOOD SWINGS, EMOTIONAL (E)		CALM, NEUTRAL, DAY-TO-DAY (C)		ANXIOUS, DEPRESSED, STRESSED. (S)		HAPPY, ENERGETIC. (H)		Use this key to track your mood changes below.	
MOOD										
BLOATING										

MEDICATION & SUPPLEMENT TRACKING & DOSE

CYCLE DAY	21	22	23	24	25	26	27	28	29	30
MEDICATION NAME EXAMPLE	DOSE	N/A								

FERTILITY TRACKER

CYCLE DAY	31	32	33	34	35	36	37	38	39	40
DATE										
DAY OF THE WEEK										
INTERCOURSE Y/N										
WAKING TEMP.										
CERVICAL FLUID Y/N										
CERVICAL FLUID KEY FOR TYPES	EGGWHITE LIKE SLIPPERY, STRETCHY (E)		CREAMY OPAQUE, MILKY, LOTION-LIKE (C)		STICKY RUBBERY, CRUMBLES, CEMENT (S)		BLEEDING (B)		Use this key to track your cervical fluid changes below.	
CERVICAL FLUID TYPE										
OVULATION Y/N										
OVULATION PAIN Y/N										
LH SPIKE										
STRESS Y/N										
ILLNESS Y/N										
SORE BREASTS Y/N										
CRAMPING										
MOOD TYPE KEY	HORMONAL, MOOD SWINGS, EMOTIONAL (E)		CALM, NEUTRAL, DAY-TO-DAY (C)		ANXIOUS, DEPRESSED, STRESSED. (S)		HAPPY, ENERGETIC. (H)		Use this key to track your mood changes below.	
MOOD										
BLOATING										

MEDICATION & SUPPLEMENT TRACKING & DOSE

CYCLE DAY	31	32	33	34	35	36	37	38	39	40
MEDICATION NAME EXAMPLE	DOSE	N/A								

MEDICATION LOG   WEEK_____ CYCLE _____ DATE _____

CYCLE DAY / MEDICATION	1	2	3	4	5	6	7	8	9	10
MEDICATION NAME EXAMPLE	DOSE TIMESTAMP									

CYCLE DAY / MEDICATION	11	12	13	14	15	16	17	18	19	20

MEDICATION LOG   WEEK_____ CYCLE _____ DATE _____

CYCLE DAY / MEDICATION	21	22	23	24	25	26	27	28	29	30
MEDICATION NAME EXAMPLE	DOSE TIMESTAMP									

CYCLE DAY / MEDICATION	31	32	33	34	35	36	37	38	39	40

RESULTS, HORMONE AND SYMPTOM LOG   WEEK_____ CYCLE _____ DATE _____

CYCLE DAY RESULTS & SYMPTOMS	1	2	3	4	5	6	7	8	9	10
DATE										
BASAL TEMP										
LH										
PROGESTERONE										
OESTROGEN										
ENDOTHICKNESS										
FOLLICLES RIGHT # & SIZE										
FOLLICLES LEFT # & SIZE										
FILL IN YOUR OWN										

CYCLE DAY RESULTS & SYMPTOMS	11	12	13	14	15	16	17	18	19	20
DATE										
BASAL TEMP										
LH										
PROGESTERONE										
OESTROGEN										
ENDOTHICKNESS										
FOLLICLES RIGHT # & SIZE										
FOLLICLES LEFT # & SIZE										
FILL IN YOUR OWN										

RESULTS, HORMONE AND SYMPTOM LOG   WEEK_____ CYCLE _____ DATE _____

CYCLE DAY / RESULTS & SYMPTOMS	21	22	23	24	25	26	27	28	29	30
DATE										
BASAL TEMP										
LH										
PROGESTERONE										
OESTROGEN										
ENDOTHICKNESS										
FOLLICLES RIGHT # & SIZE										
FOLLICLES LEFT # & SIZE										
FILL IN YOUR OWN										

CYCLE DAY / RESULTS & SYMPTOMS	31	32	33	34	35	36	37	38	39	40
DATE										
BASAL TEMP										
LH										
PROGESTERONE										
OESTROGEN										
ENDOTHICKNESS										
FOLLICLES RIGHT # & SIZE										
FOLLICLES LEFT # & SIZE										
FILL IN YOUR OWN										

SYMPTOM TRACKER

DATE	TIME	DURATION	DESCRIPTION
DATE	TIME	DURATION	DESCRIPTION

WRITE YOUR BLOOD, URINE AND OTHER TEST RESULTS

TEST	RESULT	RESULT	RESULT	RESULT

MONTH:

1 2 3 4 5 6 7 8 9 10

11 12 13 14 15 16 17 18 19

20 21 22 23 24 25 26 27 28

29 30 31

MONTH:

1 2 3 4 5 6 7 8 9 10

11 12 13 14 15 16 17 18 19

20 21 22 23 24 25 26 27 28

29 30 31

APPOINTMENT, TREATMENT AND PLANNING CALENDAR

CIRCLE GOOD DAYS PUT AN X THROUGH BAD DAYS FOR AN OVERALL VIEW OF IMPROVEMENTS

MONTH:

1	2	3	4	5	6	7
8	9	10	11	12	13	14
15	16	17	18	19	20	21
22	23	24	25	26	27	28
29	30	31				

NOTES:

_____

_____

_____

_____

_____

_____

_____

MONTH:

1	2	3	4	5	6	7
8	9	10	11	12	13	14
15	16	17	18	19	20	21
22	23	24	25	26	27	28
29	30	31				

MONTH:

1	2	3	4	5	6	7
8	9	10	11	12	13	14
15	16	17	18	19	20	21
22	23	24	25	26	27	28
29	30	31				

MONTH:

1	2	3	4	5	6	7
8	9	10	11	12	13	14
15	16	17	18	19	20	21
22	23	24	25	26	27	28
29	30	31				

NOTES:

_____

_____

_____

_____

_____

_____

_____

_____

MONTH:

1	2	3	4	5	6	7
8	9	10	11	12	13	14
15	16	17	18	19	20	21
22	23	24	25	26	27	28
29	30	31				

MONTH:

1	2	3	4	5	6	7
8	9	10	11	12	13	14
15	16	17	18	19	20	21
22	23	24	25	26	27	28
29	30	31				

USE FOR TRANSFER DAYS, THE TWO WEEK WAIT, CYCLE TRACKING, DOCTORS APPOINTMENTS OR JUST "GOOD DAYS" VS "BAD DAYS IN YOUR JOURNEY.

APPOINTMENT, TREATMENT AND PLANNING CALENDAR

CIRCLE GOOD DAYS PUT AN X THROUGH BAD DAYS FOR AN OVERALL VIEW OF IMPROVEMENTS

MONTH:

1 2 3 4 5 6 7
8 9 10 11 12 13 14
15 16 17 18 19 20 21
22 23 24 25 26 27 28
29 30 31

MONTH:

1 2 3 4 5 6 7
8 9 10 11 12 13 14
15 16 17 18 19 20 21
22 23 24 25 26 27 28
29 30 31

MONTH:

1 2 3 4 5 6 7
8 9 10 11 12 13 14
15 16 17 18 19 20 21
22 23 24 25 26 27 28
29 30 31

NOTES:

_____
_____
_____
_____
_____
_____
_____

MONTH:

1 2 3 4 5 6 7
8 9 10 11 12 13 14
15 16 17 18 19 20 21
22 23 24 25 26 27 28
29 30 31

MONTH:

1 2 3 4 5 6 7
8 9 10 11 12 13 14
15 16 17 18 19 20 21
22 23 24 25 26 27 28
29 30 31

MONTH:

1 2 3 4 5 6 7
8 9 10 11 12 13 14
15 16 17 18 19 20 21
22 23 24 25 26 27 28
29 30 31

NOTES:

_____
_____
_____
_____
_____
_____
_____

USE FOR TRANSFER DAYS, THE TWO WEEK WAIT, CYCLE TRACKING, DOCTORS APPOINTMENTS OR JUST "GOOD DAYS" VS "BAD DAYS IN YOUR JOURNEY.

MONTH:

1 2 3 4 5 6 7 8 9 10

11 12 13 14 15 16 17 18 19

20 21 22 23 24 25 26 27 28

29 30 31

DAILY ENERGY VS MOOD TRACKER

TRACK YOUR DAILY ENERGY AND MOOD, AS WELL AS DETAILS IN THE NOTES SECTION TO SPOT TRIGGERS.

100

75

50

25

0

| MONDAY | TUESDAY | WEDNESDAY | THURSDAY | FRIDAY | SATURDAY | SUNDAY |

FATIGUE/ENERGY

MOOD/ ANXIETYY

_____
_____
_____
_____
_____
_____
_____
_____
_____
_____
_____
_____
_____
_____
_____
_____
_____
_____
_____
_____

FERTILITY TRACKER

CYCLE DAY	1	2	3	4	5	6	7	8	9	10
DATE										
DAY OF THE WEEK										
INTERCOURSE Y/N										
WAKING TEMP.										
CERVICAL FLUID Y/N										
CERVICAL FLUID KEY FOR TYPES	EGGWHITE LIKE SLIPPERY, STRETCHY (E)		CREAMY OPAQUE, MILKY, LOTION-LIKE (C)		STICKY RUBBERY, CRUMBLES, CEMENT (S)		BLEEDING (B)		Use this key to track your cervical fluid changes below.	
CERVICAL FLUID TYPE										
OVULATION Y/N										
OVULATION PAIN Y/N										
LH SPIKE										
STRESS Y/N										
ILLNESS Y/N										
SORE BREASTS Y/N										
CRAMPING										
MOOD TYPE KEY	HORMONAL, MOOD SWINGS, EMOTIONAL (E)		CALM, NEUTRAL, DAY-TO-DAY (C)		ANXIOUS, DEPRESSED, STRESSED. (S)		HAPPY, ENERGETIC. (H)		Use this key to track your mood changes below.	
MOOD										
BLOATING										

MEDICATION & SUPPLEMENT TRACKING & DOSE

CYCLE DAY	1	2	3	4	5	6	7	8	9	10
MEDICATION NAME EXAMPLE	DOSE	N/A								

FERTILITY TRACKER

CYCLE DAY	11	12	13	14	15	16	17	18	19	20
DATE										
DAY OF THE WEEK										
INTERCOURSE Y/N										
WAKING TEMP.										
CERVICAL FLUID Y/N										
CERVICAL FLUID KEY FOR TYPES	EGGWHITE LIKE SLIPPERY, STRETCHY (E)		CREAMY OPAQUE, MILKY, LOTION-LIKE (C)		STICKY RUBBERY, CRUMBLES, CEMENT (S)		BLEEDING (B)		Use this key to track your cervical fluid changes below.	
CERVICAL FLUID TYPE										
OVULATION Y/N										
OVULATION PAIN Y/N										
LH SPIKE										
STRESS Y/N										
ILLNESS Y/N										
SORE BREASTS Y/N										
CRAMPING										
MOOD TYPE KEY	HORMONAL, MOOD SWINGS, EMOTIONAL (E)		CALM, NEUTRAL, DAY-TO-DAY (C)		ANXIOUS, DEPRESSED, STRESSED. (S)		HAPPY, ENERGETIC. (H)		Use this key to track your mood changes below.	
MOOD										
BLOATING										

MEDICATION & SUPPLEMENT TRACKING & DOSE

CYCLE DAY	11	12	13	14	15	16	17	18	19	20
MEDICATION NAME EXAMPLE	DOSE	N/A								

FERTILITY TRACKER

CYCLE DAY	21	22	23	24	25	26	27	28	29	30
DATE										
DAY OF THE WEEK										
INTERCOURSE Y/N										
WAKING TEMP.										
CERVICAL FLUID Y/N										
CERVICAL FLUID KEY FOR TYPES	EGGWHITE LIKE (E) SLIPPERY, STRETCHY		CREAMY (C) OPAQUE, MILKY, LOTION-LIKE		STICKY (S) RUBBERY, CRUMBLES, CEMENT		BLEEDING (B)		Use this key to track your cervical fluid changes below.	
CERVICAL FLUID TYPE										
OVULATION Y/N										
OVULATION PAIN Y/N										
LH SPIKE										
STRESS Y/N										
ILLNESS Y/N										
SORE BREASTS Y/N										
CRAMPING										
MOOD TYPE KEY	HORMONAL, (E) MOOD SWINGS, EMOTIONAL		CALM, (C) NEUTRAL, DAY-TO-DAY		ANXIOUS, (S) DEPRESSED, STRESSED.		HAPPY, (H) ENERGETIC.		Use this key to track your mood changes below.	
MOOD										
BLOATING										

MEDICATION & SUPPLEMENT TRACKING & DOSE

CYCLE DAY	21	22	23	24	25	26	27	28	29	30
MEDICATION NAME EXAMPLE	DOSE	N/A								

FERTILITY TRACKER

CYCLE DAY	31	32	33	34	35	36	37	38	39	40
DATE										
DAY OF THE WEEK										
INTERCOURSE Y/N										
WAKING TEMP.										
CERVICAL FLUID Y/N										
CERVICAL FLUID KEY FOR TYPES	EGGWHITE LIKE SLIPPERY, STRETCHY (E)		CREAMY OPAQUE, MILKY, LOTION-LIKE (C)		STICKY RUBBERY, CRUMBLES, CEMENT (S)		BLEEDING (B)		Use this key to track your cervical fluid changes below.	
CERVICAL FLUID TYPE										
OVULATION Y/N										
OVULATION PAIN Y/N										
LH SPIKE										
STRESS Y/N										
ILLNESS Y/N										
SORE BREASTS Y/N										
CRAMPING										
MOOD TYPE KEY	HORMONAL, MOOD SWINGS, EMOTIONAL (E)		CALM, NEUTRAL, DAY-TO-DAY (C)		ANXIOUS, DEPRESSED, STRESSED. (S)		HAPPY, ENERGETIC. (H)		Use this key to track your mood changes below.	
MOOD										
BLOATING										

MEDICATION & SUPPLEMENT TRACKING & DOSE

CYCLE DAY	31	32	33	34	35	36	37	38	39	40
MEDICATION NAME EXAMPLE	DOSE	N/A								

MEDICATION LOG   WEEK_____ CYCLE _____ DATE _____

CYCLE DAY / MEDICATION	1	2	3	4	5	6	7	8	9	10
MEDICATION NAME EXAMPLE	DOSE TIMESTAMP									

CYCLE DAY / MEDICATION	11	12	13	14	15	16	17	18	19	20

CYCLE DAY MEDICATION	21	22	23	24	25	26	27	28	29	30
MEDICATION NAME EXAMPLE	DOSE TIMESTAMP									

CYCLE DAY MEDICATION	31	32	33	34	35	36	37	38	39	40

RESULTS, HORMONE AND SYMPTOM LOG   WEEK_____ CYCLE _____ DATE _____

CYCLE DAY RESULTS & SYMPTOMS	1	2	3	4	5	6	7	8	9	10
DATE										
BASAL TEMP										
LH										
PROGESTERONE										
OESTROGEN										
ENDOTHICKNESS										
FOLLICLES RIGHT # & SIZE										
FOLLICLES LEFT # & SIZE										
FILL IN YOUR OWN										

CYCLE DAY RESULTS & SYMPTOMS	11	12	13	14	15	16	17	18	19	20
DATE										
BASAL TEMP										
LH										
PROGESTERONE										
OESTROGEN										
ENDOTHICKNESS										
FOLLICLES RIGHT # & SIZE										
FOLLICLES LEFT # & SIZE										
FILL IN YOUR OWN										

RESULTS, HORMONE AND SYMPTOM LOG   WEEK_____ CYCLE _____ DATE _____

CYCLE DAY / RESULTS & SYMPTOMS	21	22	23	24	25	26	27	28	29	30
DATE										
BASAL TEMP										
LH										
PROGESTERONE										
OESTROGEN										
ENDOTHICKNESS										
FOLLICLES RIGHT # & SIZE										
FOLLICLES LEFT # & SIZE										
FILL IN YOUR OWN										

CYCLE DAY / RESULTS & SYMPTOMS	31	32	33	34	35	36	37	38	39	40
DATE										
BASAL TEMP										
LH										
PROGESTERONE										
OESTROGEN										
ENDOTHICKNESS										
FOLLICLES RIGHT # & SIZE										
FOLLICLES LEFT # & SIZE										
FILL IN YOUR OWN										

WRITE YOUR BLOOD, URINE AND OTHER TEST RESULTS

TEST	RESULT	RESULT	RESULT	RESULT

SYMPTOM TRACKER

DATE	TIME	DURATION	DESCRIPTION

MONTH:

1 2 3 4 5 6 7 8 9 10

11 12 13 14 15 16 17 18 19

20 21 22 23 24 25 26 27 28

29 30 31

MONTH:

1 2 3 4 5 6 7 8 9 10

11 12 13 14 15 16 17 18 19

20 21 22 23 24 25 26 27 28

29 30 31

MONTH:

1 2 3 4 5 6 7 8 9 10

11 12 13 14 15 16 17 18 19

20 21 22 23 24 25 26 27 28

29 30 31

One Minute Meditation

Breathe in through your nose.

Breathe out through your mouth.

Feel air in the depths of your lungs
as you breathe in again.

As you breathe out feel tension
release from your body.

Repeat 3x.

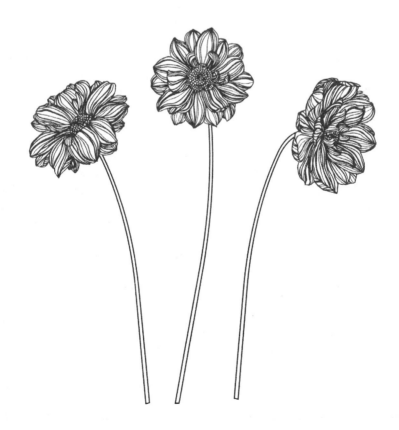

WHAT BODY PART ARE YOU GRATEFUL FOR?

ANSWER THESE QUESTIONS TO BREAK OUT OF NEGATIVE
THOUGHT PATTERNS AND REFOCUS ON THE THINGS THAT MAKE
YOU HAPPY AND GRATEFUL.

DAILY ENERGY VS MOOD TRACKER

TRACK YOUR DAILY ENERGY AND MOOD, AS WELL AS DETAILS IN THE NOTES SECTION TO SPOT TRIGGERS.

100

75

50

25

0

| MONDAY | TUESDAY | WEDNESDAY | THURSDAY | FRIDAY | SATURDAY | SUNDAY |

FATIGUE/ENERGY

MOOD/ ANXIETYY

_____

_____

_____

_____

_____

_____

_____

_____

_____

_____

_____

_____

_____

_____

_____

_____

_____

_____

FERTILITY TRACKER

CYCLE DAY	1	2	3	4	5	6	7	8	9	10
DATE										
DAY OF THE WEEK										
INTERCOURSE Y/N										
WAKING TEMP.										
CERVICAL FLUID Y/N										
CERVICAL FLUID KEY FOR TYPES	EGGWHITE LIKE SLIPPERY, STRETCHY (E)		CREAMY OPAQUE, MILKY, LOTION-LIKE (C)		STICKY RUBBERY, CRUMBLES, CEMENT (S)		BLEEDING (B)		Use this key to track your cervical fluid changes below.	
CERVICAL FLUID TYPE										
OVULATION Y/N										
OVULATION PAIN Y/N										
LH SPIKE										
STRESS Y/N										
ILLNESS Y/N										
SORE BREASTS Y/N										
CRAMPING										
MOOD TYPE KEY	HORMONAL, MOOD SWINGS, EMOTIONAL (E)		CALM, NEUTRAL, DAY-TO-DAY (C)		ANXIOUS, DEPRESSED, STRESSED. (S)		HAPPY, ENERGETIC. (H)		Use this key to track your mood changes below.	
MOOD										
BLOATING										

MEDICATION & SUPPLEMENT TRACKING & DOSE

CYCLE DAY	1	2	3	4	5	6	7	8	9	10
MEDICATION NAME EXAMPLE	DOSE	N/A								

FERTILITY TRACKER

CYCLE DAY	11	12	13	14	15	16	17	18	19	20
DATE										
DAY OF THE WEEK										
INTERCOURSE Y/N										
WAKING TEMP.										
CERVICAL FLUID Y/N										
CERVICAL FLUID KEY FOR TYPES	EGGWHITE LIKE (E) SLIPPERY, STRETCHY		CREAMY (C) OPAQUE, MILKY, LOTION-LIKE		STICKY (S) RUBBERY, CRUMBLES, CEMENT		BLEEDING (B)		Use this key to track your cervical fluid changes below.	
CERVICAL FLUID TYPE										
OVULATION Y/N										
OVULATION PAIN Y/N										
LH SPIKE										
STRESS Y/N										
ILLNESS Y/N										
SORE BREASTS Y/N										
CRAMPING										
MOOD TYPE KEY	HORMONAL, (E) MOOD SWINGS, EMOTIONAL		CALM, (C) NEUTRAL, DAY-TO-DAY		ANXIOUS, (S) DEPRESSED, STRESSED.		HAPPY, (H) ENERGETIC.		Use this key to track your mood changes below.	
MOOD										
BLOATING										

MEDICATION & SUPPLEMENT TRACKING & DOSE

CYCLE DAY	11	12	13	14	15	16	17	18	19	20
MEDICATION NAME EXAMPLE	DOSE	N/A								

FERTILITY TRACKER

CYCLE DAY	21	22	23	24	25	26	27	28	29	30
DATE										
DAY OF THE WEEK										
INTERCOURSE Y/N										
WAKING TEMP.										
CERVICAL FLUID Y/N										
CERVICAL FLUID KEY FOR TYPES	EGGWHITE LIKE SLIPPERY, STRETCHY (E)		CREAMY OPAQUE, MILKY, LOTION-LIKE (C)		STICKY RUBBERY, CRUMBLES, CEMENT (S)		BLEEDING (B)		Use this key to track your cervical fluid changes below.	
CERVICAL FLUID TYPE										
OVULATION Y/N										
OVULATION PAIN Y/N										
LH SPIKE										
STRESS Y/N										
ILLNESS Y/N										
SORE BREASTS Y/N										
CRAMPING										
MOOD TYPE KEY	HORMONAL, MOOD SWINGS, EMOTIONAL (E)		CALM, NEUTRAL, DAY-TO-DAY (C)		ANXIOUS, DEPRESSED, STRESSED. (S)		HAPPY, ENERGETIC. (H)		Use this key to track your mood changes below.	
MOOD										
BLOATING										

MEDICATION & SUPPLEMENT TRACKING & DOSE

CYCLE DAY	21	22	23	24	25	26	27	28	29	30
MEDICATION NAME EXAMPLE	DOSE	N/A								

FERTILITY TRACKER

CYCLE DAY	31	32	33	34	35	36	37	38	39	40
DATE										
DAY OF THE WEEK										
INTERCOURSE Y/N										
WAKING TEMP.										
CERVICAL FLUID Y/N										
CERVICAL FLUID KEY FOR TYPES	EGGWHITE LIKE SLIPPERY, STRETCHY (E)		CREAMY OPAQUE, MILKY, LOTION-LIKE (C)		STICKY RUBBERY, CRUMBLES, CEMENT (S)		BLEEDING (B)		Use this key to track your cervical fluid changes below.	
CERVICAL FLUID TYPE										
OVULATION Y/N										
OVULATION PAIN Y/N										
LH SPIKE										
STRESS Y/N										
ILLNESS Y/N										
SORE BREASTS Y/N										
CRAMPING										
MOOD TYPE KEY	HORMONAL, MOOD SWINGS, EMOTIONAL (E)		CALM, NEUTRAL, DAY-TO-DAY (C)		ANXIOUS, DEPRESSED, STRESSED. (S)		HAPPY, ENERGETIC. (H)		Use this key to track your mood changes below.	
MOOD										
BLOATING										

MEDICATION & SUPPLEMENT TRACKING & DOSE

CYCLE DAY	31	32	33	34	35	36	37	38	39	40
MEDICATION NAME EXAMPLE	DOSE	N/A								

MEDICATION LOG   WEEK_____ CYCLE _____ DATE _____

CYCLE DAY / MEDICATION	1	2	3	4	5	6	7	8	9	10
MEDICATION NAME EXAMPLE	DOSE TIMESTAMP									

CYCLE DAY / MEDICATION	11	12	13	14	15	16	17	18	19	20

MEDICATION LOG   WEEK_____ CYCLE _____ DATE _____

CYCLE DAY / MEDICATION	21	22	23	24	25	26	27	28	29	30
MEDICATION NAME EXAMPLE	DOSE TIMESTAMP									

CYCLE DAY / MEDICATION	31	32	33	34	35	36	37	38	39	40

RESULTS, HORMONE AND SYMPTOM LOG WEEK_____ CYCLE _____ DATE _____

CYCLE DAY RESULTS & SYMPTOMS	1	2	3	4	5	6	7	8	9	10
DATE										
BASAL TEMP										
LH										
PROGESTERONE										
OESTROGEN										
ENDOTHICKNESS										
FOLLICLES RIGHT # & SIZE										
FOLLICLES LEFT # & SIZE										
FILL IN YOUR OWN										

CYCLE DAY RESULTS & SYMPTOMS	11	12	13	14	15	16	17	18	19	20
DATE										
BASAL TEMP										
LH										
PROGESTERONE										
OESTROGEN										
ENDOTHICKNESS										
FOLLICLES RIGHT # & SIZE										
FOLLICLES LEFT # & SIZE										
FILL IN YOUR OWN										

RESULTS, HORMONE AND SYMPTOM LOG   WEEK_____ CYCLE _____ DATE _____

CYCLE DAY / RESULTS & SYMPTOMS	21	22	23	24	25	26	27	28	29	30
DATE										
BASAL TEMP										
LH										
PROGESTERONE										
OESTROGEN										
ENDOTHICKNESS										
FOLLICLES RIGHT # & SIZE										
FOLLICLES LEFT # & SIZE										
FILL IN YOUR OWN										

CYCLE DAY / RESULTS & SYMPTOMS	31	32	33	34	35	36	37	38	39	40
DATE										
BASAL TEMP										
LH										
PROGESTERONE										
OESTROGEN										
ENDOTHICKNESS										
FOLLICLES RIGHT # & SIZE										
FOLLICLES LEFT # & SIZE										
FILL IN YOUR OWN										

SYMPTOM TRACKER

DATE	TIME	DURATION	DESCRIPTION

DOCTORS APPOINTMENTS TIME SHEET

DATE	TIME	DOCTOR & LOCATION	REASON & NOTES

EMERGENCY & DOCTORS CONTACTS

_____
_____
_____
_____
_____
_____

MONTH:

1 2 3 4 5 6 7 8 9 10

11 12 13 14 15 16 17 18 19

20 21 22 23 24 25 26 27 28

29 30 31

MONTH:

1 2 3 4 5 6 7 8 9 10

11 12 13 14 15 16 17 18 19

20 21 22 23 24 25 26 27 28

29 30 31

MONTH:

1 2 3 4 5 6 7 8 9 10

11 12 13 14 15 16 17 18 19

20 21 22 23 24 25 26 27 28

29 30 31

WHAT I HOPE IS YET TO COME...

ANSWER THESE QUESTIONS TO BREAK OUT OF NEGATIVE
THOUGHT PATTERNS AND REFOCUS ON THE THINGS THAT MAKE
YOU HAPPY AND GRATEFUL.

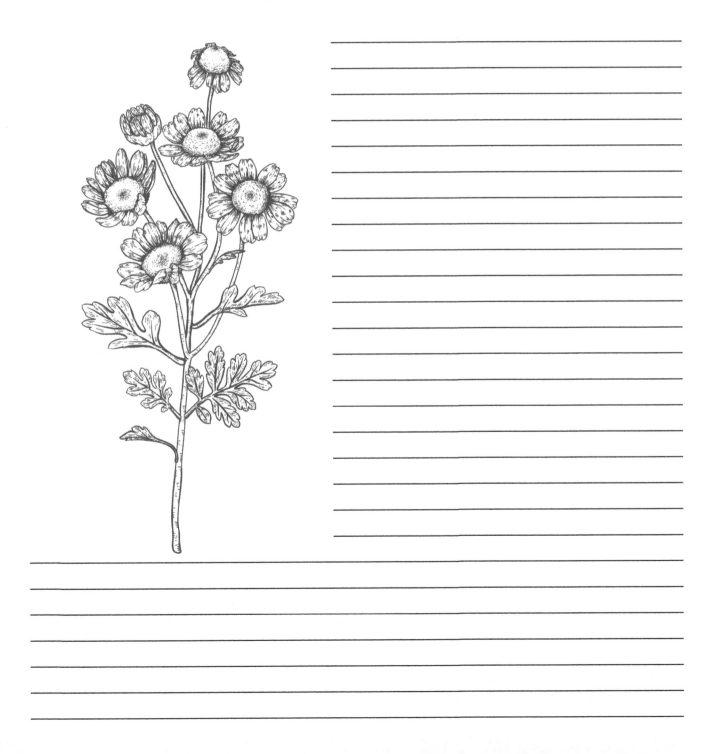

DAILY ENERGY VS MOOD TRACKER

TRACK YOUR DAILY ENERGY AND MOOD, AS WELL AS DETAILS IN THE NOTES SECTION TO SPOT TRIGGERS.

100

75

50

25

0   MONDAY   TUESDAY   WEDNESDAY   THURSDAY   FRIDAY   SATURDAY   SUNDAY

FATIGUE/ENERGY   MOOD/ ANXIETYY

FERTILITY TRACKER

CYCLE DAY	1	2	3	4	5	6	7	8	9	10
DATE										
DAY OF THE WEEK										
INTERCOURSE Y/N										
WAKING TEMP.										
CERVICAL FLUID Y/N										
CERVICAL FLUID KEY FOR TYPES	EGGWHITE LIKE SLIPPERY, STRETCHY (E)		CREAMY OPAQUE, MILKY, LOTION-LIKE (C)		STICKY RUBBERY, CRUMBLES, CEMENT (S)		BLEEDING (B)		Use this key to track your cervical fluid changes below.	
CERVICAL FLUID TYPE										
OVULATION Y/N										
OVULATION PAIN Y/N										
LH SPIKE										
STRESS Y/N										
ILLNESS Y/N										
SORE BREASTS Y/N										
CRAMPING										
MOOD TYPE KEY	HORMONAL, MOOD SWINGS, EMOTIONAL (E)		CALM, NEUTRAL, DAY-TO-DAY (C)		ANXIOUS, DEPRESSED, STRESSED. (S)		HAPPY, ENERGETIC. (H)		Use this key to track your mood changes below.	
MOOD										
BLOATING										

MEDICATION & SUPPLEMENT TRACKING & DOSE

CYCLE DAY	1	2	3	4	5	6	7	8	9	10
MEDICATION NAME EXAMPLE	DOSE	N/A								

FERTILITY TRACKER

CYCLE DAY	11	12	13	14	15	16	17	18	19	20
DATE										
DAY OF THE WEEK										
INTERCOURSE Y/N										
WAKING TEMP.										
CERVICAL FLUID Y/N										
CERVICAL FLUID KEY FOR TYPES	EGGWHITE LIKE, SLIPPERY, STRETCHY (E)		CREAMY OPAQUE, MILKY, LOTION-LIKE (C)		STICKY RUBBERY, CRUMBLES, CEMENT (S)		BLEEDING (B)		Use this key to track your cervical fluid changes below.	
CERVICAL FLUID TYPE										
OVULATION Y/N										
OVULATION PAIN Y/N										
LH SPIKE										
STRESS Y/N										
ILLNESS Y/N										
SORE BREASTS Y/N										
CRAMPING										
MOOD TYPE KEY	HORMONAL, MOOD SWINGS, EMOTIONAL (E)		CALM, NEUTRAL, DAY-TO-DAY (C)		ANXIOUS, DEPRESSED, STRESSED. (S)		HAPPY, ENERGETIC. (H)		Use this key to track your mood changes below.	
MOOD										
BLOATING										

MEDICATION & SUPPLEMENT TRACKING & DOSE

CYCLE DAY	11	12	13	14	15	16	17	18	19	20
MEDICATION NAME EXAMPLE	DOSE	N/A								

FERTILITY TRACKER

CYCLE DAY	21	22	23	24	25	26	27	28	29	30
DATE										
DAY OF THE WEEK										
INTERCOURSE Y/N										
WAKING TEMP.										
CERVICAL FLUID Y/N										
CERVICAL FLUID KEY FOR TYPES	EGGWHITE LIKE (E) SLIPPERY, STRETCHY		CREAMY (C) OPAQUE, MILKY, LOTION-LIKE		STICKY (S) RUBBERY, CRUMBLES, CEMENT		BLEEDING (B)		Use this key to track your cervical fluid changes below.	
CERVICAL FLUID TYPE										
OVULATION Y/N										
OVULATION PAIN Y/N										
LH SPIKE										
STRESS Y/N										
ILLNESS Y/N										
SORE BREASTS Y/N										
CRAMPING										
MOOD TYPE KEY	HORMONAL, (E) MOOD SWINGS, EMOTIONAL		CALM, (C) NEUTRAL, DAY-TO-DAY		ANXIOUS, (S) DEPRESSED, STRESSED.		HAPPY, (H) ENERGETIC.		Use this key to track your mood changes below.	
MOOD										
BLOATING										

MEDICATION & SUPPLEMENT TRACKING & DOSE

CYCLE DAY	21	22	23	24	25	26	27	28	29	30
MEDICATION NAME EXAMPLE	DOSE	N/A								

FERTILITY TRACKER

CYCLE DAY	31	32	33	34	35	36	37	38	39	40
DATE										
DAY OF THE WEEK										
INTERCOURSE Y/N										
WAKING TEMP.										
CERVICAL FLUID Y/N										
CERVICAL FLUID KEY FOR TYPES	EGGWHITE LIKE SLIPPERY, STRETCHY (E)	CREAMY OPAQUE, MILKY, LOTION-LIKE (C)	STICKY RUBBERY, CRUMBLES, CEMENT (S)		BLEEDING (B)				Use this key to track your cervical fluid changes below.	
CERVICAL FLUID TYPE										
OVULATION Y/N										
OVULATION PAIN Y/N										
LH SPIKE										
STRESS Y/N										
ILLNESS Y/N										
SORE BREASTS Y/N										
CRAMPING										
MOOD TYPE KEY	HORMONAL, MOOD SWINGS, EMOTIONAL (E)	CALM, NEUTRAL, DAY-TO-DAY (C)	ANXIOUS, DEPRESSED, STRESSED. (S)		HAPPY, ENERGETIC. (H)				Use this key to track your mood changes below.	
MOOD										
BLOATING										

MEDICATION & SUPPLEMENT TRACKING & DOSE

CYCLE DAY	31	32	33	34	35	36	37	38	39	40
MEDICATION NAME EXAMPLE	DOSE	N/A								

MEDICATION LOG   WEEK_____   CYCLE _____   DATE _____

CYCLE DAY / MEDICATION	1	2	3	4	5	6	7	8	9	10
MEDICATION NAME EXAMPLE	DOSE TIMESTAMP									

CYCLE DAY / MEDICATION	11	12	13	14	15	16	17	18	19	20

CYCLE DAY / MEDICATION	21	22	23	24	25	26	27	28	29	30
MEDICATION NAME EXAMPLE	DOSE TIMESTAMP									

CYCLE DAY / MEDICATION	31	32	33	34	35	36	37	38	39	40

RESULTS, HORMONE AND SYMPTOM LOG   WEEK_____ CYCLE _____ DATE _____

CYCLE DAY RESULTS & SYMPTOMS	1	2	3	4	5	6	7	8	9	10
DATE										
BASAL TEMP										
LH										
PROGESTERONE										
OESTROGEN										
ENDOTHICKNESS										
FOLLICLES RIGHT # & SIZE										
FOLLICLES LEFT # & SIZE										
FILL IN YOUR OWN										

CYCLE DAY RESULTS & SYMPTOMS	11	12	13	14	15	16	17	18	19	20
DATE										
BASAL TEMP										
LH										
PROGESTERONE										
OESTROGEN										
ENDOTHICKNESS										
FOLLICLES RIGHT # & SIZE										
FOLLICLES LEFT # & SIZE										
FILL IN YOUR OWN										

RESULTS, HORMONE AND SYMPTOM LOG   WEEK_____ CYCLE _____ DATE _____

CYCLE DAY / RESULTS & SYMPTOMS	21	22	23	24	25	26	27	28	29	30
DATE										
BASAL TEMP										
LH										
PROGESTERONE										
OESTROGEN										
ENDOTHICKNESS										
FOLLICLES RIGHT # & SIZE										
FOLLICLES LEFT # & SIZE										
FILL IN YOUR OWN										

CYCLE DAY / RESULTS & SYMPTOMS	31	32	33	34	35	36	37	38	39	40
DATE										
BASAL TEMP										
LH										
PROGESTERONE										
OESTROGEN										
ENDOTHICKNESS										
FOLLICLES RIGHT # & SIZE										
FOLLICLES LEFT # & SIZE										
FILL IN YOUR OWN										

EVEN MIRACLES
TAKE SOME TIME.

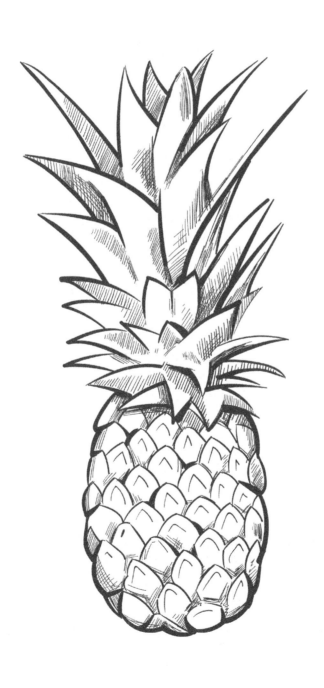

MONTH:

1 2 3 4 5 6 7 8 9 10

11 12 13 14 15 16 17 18 19

20 21 22 23 24 25 26 27 28

29 30 31

MONTH:

1 2 3 4 5 6 7 8 9 10

11 12 13 14 15 16 17 18 19

20 21 22 23 24 25 26 27 28

29 30 31

MONTH:

1 2 3 4 5 6 7 8 9 10

11 12 13 14 15 16 17 18 19

20 21 22 23 24 25 26 27 28

29 30 31

DAILY ENERGY VS MOOD TRACKER

TRACK YOUR DAILY ENERGY AND MOOD, AS WELL AS DETAILS IN THE NOTES SECTION TO SPOT TRIGGERS.

	100						
	75						
	50						
	25						
	0	MONDAY	TUESDAY	WEDNESDAY	THURSDAY	FRIDAY	SATURDAY	SUNDAY

FATIGUE/ENERGY

MOOD/ ANXIETYY

_____
_____
_____
_____
_____
_____
_____
_____
_____
_____
_____
_____
_____
_____
_____
_____
_____
_____
_____

FERTILITY TRACKER

CYCLE DAY	1	2	3	4	5	6	7	8	9	10
DATE										
DAY OF THE WEEK										
INTERCOURSE Y/N										
WAKING TEMP.										
CERVICAL FLUID Y/N										
CERVICAL FLUID KEY FOR TYPES	EGGWHITE LIKE SLIPPERY, STRETCHY (E)		CREAMY OPAQUE, MILKY, LOTION-LIKE (C)		STICKY RUBBERY, CRUMBLES, CEMENT (S)		BLEEDING (B)		Use this key to track your cervical fluid changes below.	
CERVICAL FLUID TYPE										
OVULATION Y/N										
OVULATION PAIN Y/N										
LH SPIKE										
STRESS Y/N										
ILLNESS Y/N										
SORE BREASTS Y/N										
CRAMPING										
MOOD TYPE KEY	HORMONAL, MOOD SWINGS, EMOTIONAL (E)		CALM, NEUTRAL, DAY-TO-DAY (C)		ANXIOUS, DEPRESSED, STRESSED. (S)		HAPPY, ENERGETIC. (H)		Use this key to track your mood changes below.	
MOOD										
BLOATING										

MEDICATION & SUPPLEMENT TRACKING & DOSE

CYCLE DAY	1	2	3	4	5	6	7	8	9	10
MEDICATION NAME EXAMPLE	DOSE	N/A								

FERTILITY TRACKER

CYCLE DAY	11	12	13	14	15	16	17	18	19	20
DATE										
DAY OF THE WEEK										
INTERCOURSE Y/N										
WAKING TEMP.										
CERVICAL FLUID Y/N										
CERVICAL FLUID KEY FOR TYPES	EGGWHITE LIKE SLIPPERY, STRETCHY (E)		CREAMY OPAQUE, MILKY, LOTION-LIKE (C)		STICKY RUBBERY, CRUMBLES, CEMENT (S)		BLEEDING (B)		Use this key to track your cervical fluid changes below.	
CERVICAL FLUID TYPE										
OVULATION Y/N										
OVULATION PAIN Y/N										
LH SPIKE										
STRESS Y/N										
ILLNESS Y/N										
SORE BREASTS Y/N										
CRAMPING										
MOOD TYPE KEY	HORMONAL, MOOD SWINGS, EMOTIONAL (E)		CALM, NEUTRAL, DAY-TO-DAY (C)		ANXIOUS, DEPRESSED, STRESSED. (S)		HAPPY, ENERGETIC. (H)		Use this key to track your mood changes below.	
MOOD										
BLOATING										

MEDICATION & SUPPLEMENT TRACKING & DOSE

CYCLE DAY	11	12	13	14	15	16	17	18	19	20
MEDICATION NAME EXAMPLE	DOSE	N/A								

FERTILITY TRACKER

CYCLE DAY	21	22	23	24	25	26	27	28	29	30
DATE										
DAY OF THE WEEK										
INTERCOURSE Y/N										
WAKING TEMP.										
CERVICAL FLUID Y/N										
CERVICAL FLUID KEY FOR TYPES	EGGWHITE LIKE (E) SLIPPERY, STRETCHY		CREAMY (C) OPAQUE, MILKY, LOTION-LIKE		STICKY (S) RUBBERY, CRUMBLES, CEMENT		BLEEDING (B)		Use this key to track your cervical fluid changes below.	
CERVICAL FLUID TYPE										
OVULATION Y/N										
OVULATION PAIN Y/N										
LH SPIKE										
STRESS Y/N										
ILLNESS Y/N										
SORE BREASTS Y/N										
CRAMPING										
MOOD TYPE KEY	HORMONAL, (E) MOOD SWINGS, EMOTIONAL		CALM, (C) NEUTRAL, DAY-TO-DAY		ANXIOUS, (S) DEPRESSED, STRESSED.		HAPPY, (H) ENERGETIC.		Use this key to track your mood changes below.	
MOOD										
BLOATING										

MEDICATION & SUPPLEMENT TRACKING & DOSE

CYCLE DAY	21	22	23	24	25	26	27	28	29	30
MEDICATION NAME EXAMPLE	DOSE	N/A								

FERTILITY TRACKER

CYCLE DAY	31	32	33	34	35	36	37	38	39	40
DATE										
DAY OF THE WEEK										
INTERCOURSE Y/N										
WAKING TEMP.										
CERVICAL FLUID Y/N										
CERVICAL FLUID KEY FOR TYPES	EGGWHITE LIKE SLIPPERY, STRETCHY (E)		CREAMY OPAQUE, MILKY, LOTION-LIKE (C)		STICKY RUBBERY, CRUMBLES. CEMENT (S)		BLEEDING (B)		Use this key to track your cervical fluid changes below.	
CERVICAL FLUID TYPE										
OVULATION Y/N										
OVULATION PAIN Y/N										
LH SPIKE										
STRESS Y/N										
ILLNESS Y/N										
SORE BREASTS Y/N										
CRAMPING										
MOOD TYPE KEY	HORMONAL, MOOD SWINGS, EMOTIONAL (E)		CALM, NEUTRAL, DAY-TO-DAY (C)		ANXIOUS, DEPRESSED, STRESSED. (S)		HAPPY, ENERGETIC. (H)		Use this key to track your mood changes below.	
MOOD										
BLOATING										

MEDICATION & SUPPLEMENT TRACKING & DOSE

CYCLE DAY	31	32	33	34	35	36	37	38	39	40
MEDICATION NAME EXAMPLE	DOSE	N/A								

MEDICATION LOG   WEEK_____   CYCLE _____   DATE _____

CYCLE DAY / MEDICATION	1	2	3	4	5	6	7	8	9	10
MEDICATION NAME EXAMPLE	DOSE TIMESTAMP									

CYCLE DAY / MEDICATION	11	12	13	14	15	16	17	18	19	20

MEDICATION LOG   WEEK_____ CYCLE _____ DATE _____

CYCLE DAY / MEDICATION	21	22	23	24	25	26	27	28	29	30
MEDICATION NAME EXAMPLE	DOSE TIMESTAMP									

CYCLE DAY / MEDICATION	31	32	33	34	35	36	37	38	39	40

CYCLE DAY RESULTS & SYMPTOMS	1	2	3	4	5	6	7	8	9	10
DATE										
BASAL TEMP										
LH										
PROGESTERONE										
OESTROGEN										
ENDOTHICKNESS										
FOLLICLES RIGHT # & SIZE										
FOLLICLES LEFT # & SIZE										
FILL IN YOUR OWN										

CYCLE DAY RESULTS & SYMPTOMS	11	12	13	14	15	16	17	18	19	20
DATE										
BASAL TEMP										
LH										
PROGESTERONE										
OESTROGEN										
ENDOTHICKNESS										
FOLLICLES RIGHT # & SIZE										
FOLLICLES LEFT # & SIZE										
FILL IN YOUR OWN										

RESULTS, HORMONE AND SYMPTOM LOG   WEEK_____ CYCLE _____ DATE _____

CYCLE DAY / RESULTS & SYMPTOMS	21	22	23	24	25	26	27	28	29	30
DATE										
BASAL TEMP										
LH										
PROGESTERONE										
OESTROGEN										
ENDOTHICKNESS										
FOLLICLES RIGHT # & SIZE										
FOLLICLES LEFT # & SIZE										
FILL IN YOUR OWN										

CYCLE DAY / RESULTS & SYMPTOMS	31	32	33	34	35	36	37	38	39	40
DATE										
BASAL TEMP										
LH										
PROGESTERONE										
OESTROGEN										
ENDOTHICKNESS										
FOLLICLES RIGHT # & SIZE										
FOLLICLES LEFT # & SIZE										
FILL IN YOUR OWN										

SYMPTOM TRACKER

DATE	TIME	DURATION	DESCRIPTION
DATE	TIME	DURATION	DESCRIPTION

DOCTORS APPOINTMENTS TIME SHEET

DATE	TIME	DOCTOR & LOCATION	REASON & NOTES

EMERGENCY & DOCTORS CONTACTS

MONTH:

1 2 3 4 5 6 7 8 9 10

11 12 13 14 15 16 17 18 19

20 21 22 23 24 25 26 27 28

29 30 31

MONTH:

1 2 3 4 5 6 7 8 9 10

11 12 13 14 15 16 17 18 19

20 21 22 23 24 25 26 27 28

29 30 31

MONTH:

1 2 3 4 5 6 7 8 9 10

11 12 13 14 15 16 17 18 19

20 21 22 23 24 25 26 27 28

29 30 31

Be gentle with yourself.

You're doing the best you can.

Take every day as it comes.

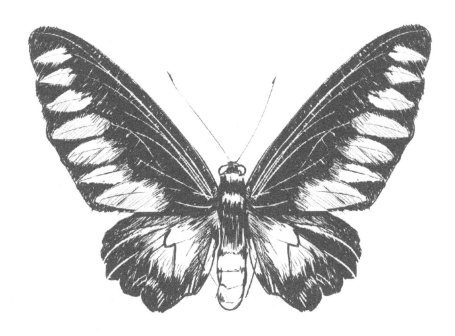

DAILY ENERGY VS MOOD TRACKER

TRACK YOUR DAILY ENERGY AND MOOD, AS WELL AS DETAILS IN THE NOTES SECTION TO SPOT TRIGGERS.

100

75

50

25

0

| MONDAY | TUESDAY | WEDNESDAY | THURSDAY | FRIDAY | SATURDAY | SUNDAY |

FATIGUE/ENERGY

MOOD/ ANXIETYY

FERTILITY TRACKER

CYCLE DAY	1	2	3	4	5	6	7	8	9	10
DATE										
DAY OF THE WEEK										
INTERCOURSE Y/N										
WAKING TEMP.										
CERVICAL FLUID Y/N										
CERVICAL FLUID KEY FOR TYPES	EGGWHITE LIKE SLIPPERY, STRETCHY (E)	CREAMY OPAQUE, MILKY, LOTION-LIKE (C)	STICKY RUBBERY, CRUMBLES, CEMENT (S)	BLEEDING (B)	Use this key to track your cervical fluid changes below.					
CERVICAL FLUID TYPE										
OVULATION Y/N										
OVULATION PAIN Y/N										
LH SPIKE										
STRESS Y/N										
ILLNESS Y/N										
SORE BREASTS Y/N										
CRAMPING										
MOOD TYPE KEY	HORMONAL, MOOD SWINGS, EMOTIONAL (E)	CALM, NEUTRAL, DAY-TO-DAY (C)	ANXIOUS, DEPRESSED, STRESSED. (S)	HAPPY, ENERGETIC. (H)	Use this key to track your mood changes below.					
MOOD										
BLOATING										

MEDICATION & SUPPLEMENT TRACKING & DOSE

CYCLE DAY	1	2	3	4	5	6	7	8	9	10
MEDICATION NAME EXAMPLE	DOSE	N/A								

FERTILITY TRACKER

CYCLE DAY	11	12	13	14	15	16	17	18	19	20
DATE										
DAY OF THE WEEK										
INTERCOURSE Y/N										
WAKING TEMP.										
CERVICAL FLUID Y/N										
CERVICAL FLUID KEY FOR TYPES	EGGWHITE LIKE (E) SLIPPERY, STRETCHY		CREAMY (C) OPAQUE, MILKY, LOTION-LIKE		STICKY (S) RUBBERY, CRUMBLES, CEMENT		BLEEDING (B)		Use this key to track your cervical fluid changes below.	
CERVICAL FLUID TYPE										
OVULATION Y/N										
OVULATION PAIN Y/N										
LH SPIKE										
STRESS Y/N										
ILLNESS Y/N										
SORE BREASTS Y/N										
CRAMPING										
MOOD TYPE KEY	HORMONAL, (E) MOOD SWINGS, EMOTIONAL		CALM, (C) NEUTRAL, DAY-TO-DAY		ANXIOUS, (S) DEPRESSED, STRESSED.		HAPPY, (H) ENERGETIC.		Use this key to track your mood changes below.	
MOOD										
BLOATING										

MEDICATION & SUPPLEMENT TRACKING & DOSE

CYCLE DAY	11	12	13	14	15	16	17	18	19	20
MEDICATION NAME EXAMPLE	DOSE	N/A								

FERTILITY TRACKER

CYCLE DAY	21	22	23	24	25	26	27	28	29	30
DATE										
DAY OF THE WEEK										
INTERCOURSE Y/N										
WAKING TEMP.										
CERVICAL FLUID Y/N										
CERVICAL FLUID KEY FOR TYPES	EGGWHITE LIKE (E) SLIPPERY, STRETCHY		CREAMY (C) OPAQUE, MILKY, LOTION-LIKE		STICKY (S) RUBBERY, CRUMBLES, CEMENT		BLEEDING (B)		Use this key to track your cervical fluid changes below.	
CERVICAL FLUID TYPE										
OVULATION Y/N										
OVULATION PAIN Y/N										
LH SPIKE										
STRESS Y/N										
ILLNESS Y/N										
SORE BREASTS Y/N										
CRAMPING										
MOOD TYPE KEY	HORMONAL, (E) MOOD SWINGS, EMOTIONAL		CALM, (C) NEUTRAL, DAY-TO-DAY		ANXIOUS, (S) DEPRESSED, STRESSED.		HAPPY, (H) ENERGETIC.		Use this key to track your mood changes below.	
MOOD										
BLOATING										

MEDICATION & SUPPLEMENT TRACKING & DOSE

CYCLE DAY	21	22	23	24	25	26	27	28	29	30
MEDICATION NAME EXAMPLE	DOSE	N/A								

FERTILITY TRACKER

CYCLE DAY	31	32	33	34	35	36	37	38	39	40
DATE										
DAY OF THE WEEK										
INTERCOURSE Y/N										
WAKING TEMP.										
CERVICAL FLUID Y/N										
CERVICAL FLUID KEY FOR TYPES	EGGWHITE LIKE (E) SLIPPERY, STRETCHY		CREAMY (C) OPAQUE, MILKY, LOTION-LIKE		STICKY (S) RUBBERY, CRUMBLES, CEMENT		BLEEDING (B)		Use this key to track your cervical fluid changes below.	
CERVICAL FLUID TYPE										
OVULATION Y/N										
OVULATION PAIN Y/N										
LH SPIKE										
STRESS Y/N										
ILLNESS Y/N										
SORE BREASTS Y/N										
CRAMPING										
MOOD TYPE KEY	HORMONAL, (E) MOOD SWINGS, EMOTIONAL		CALM, (C) NEUTRAL, DAY-TO-DAY		ANXIOUS, (S) DEPRESSED, STRESSED.		HAPPY, (H) ENERGETIC.		Use this key to track your mood changes below.	
MOOD										
BLOATING										

MEDICATION & SUPPLEMENT TRACKING & DOSE

CYCLE DAY	31	32	33	34	35	36	37	38	39	40
MEDICATION NAME EXAMPLE	DOSE	N/A								

MEDICATION LOG   WEEK_____ CYCLE _____ DATE _____

CYCLE DAY / MEDICATION	1	2	3	4	5	6	7	8	9	10
MEDICATION NAME EXAMPLE	DOSE TIMESTAMP									

CYCLE DAY / MEDICATION	11	12	13	14	15	16	17	18	19	20

MEDICATION LOG   WEEK_____ CYCLE _____ DATE _____

CYCLE DAY / MEDICATION	21	22	23	24	25	26	27	28	29	30
MEDICATION NAME EXAMPLE	DOSE TIMESTAMP									

CYCLE DAY / MEDICATION	31	32	33	34	35	36	37	38	39	40

RESULTS, HORMONE AND SYMPTOM LOG   WEEK_____ CYCLE _____ DATE _____

CYCLE DAY / RESULTS & SYMPTOMS	1	2	3	4	5	6	7	8	9	10
DATE										
BASAL TEMP										
LH										
PROGESTERONE										
OESTROGEN										
ENDOTHICKNESS										
FOLLICLES RIGHT # & SIZE										
FOLLICLES LEFT # & SIZE										
FILL IN YOUR OWN										

CYCLE DAY / RESULTS & SYMPTOMS	11	12	13	14	15	16	17	18	19	20
DATE										
BASAL TEMP										
LH										
PROGESTERONE										
OESTROGEN										
ENDOTHICKNESS										
FOLLICLES RIGHT # & SIZE										
FOLLICLES LEFT # & SIZE										
FILL IN YOUR OWN										

CYCLE DAY / RESULTS & SYMPTOMS	21	22	23	24	25	26	27	28	29	30
DATE										
BASAL TEMP										
LH										
PROGESTERONE										
OESTROGEN										
ENDOTHICKNESS										
FOLLICLES RIGHT # & SIZE										
FOLLICLES LEFT # & SIZE										
FILL IN YOUR OWN										

CYCLE DAY / RESULTS & SYMPTOMS	31	32	33	34	35	36	37	38	39	40
DATE										
BASAL TEMP										
LH										
PROGESTERONE										
OESTROGEN										
ENDOTHICKNESS										
FOLLICLES RIGHT # & SIZE										
FOLLICLES LEFT # & SIZE										
FILL IN YOUR OWN										

SYMPTOM TRACKER

DATE	TIME	DURATION	DESCRIPTION

DOCTORS APPOINTMENTS TIME SHEET

DATE	TIME	DOCTOR & LOCATION	REASON & NOTES

EMERGENCY & DOCTORS CONTACTS

MONTH:

1 2 3 4 5 6 7 8 9 10

11 12 13 14 15 16 17 18 19

20 21 22 23 24 25 26 27 28

29 30 31

MONTH:

1 2 3 4 5 6 7 8 9 10

11 12 13 14 15 16 17 18 19

20 21 22 23 24 25 26 27 28

29 30 31

MONTH:

1 2 3 4 5 6 7 8 9 10

11 12 13 14 15 16 17 18 19

20 21 22 23 24 25 26 27 28

29 30 31

WHAT GOALS DO YOU HAVE FOR YOUR HEALTH?

ANSWER THESE QUESTIONS TO BREAK OUT OF NEGATIVE
THOUGHT PATTERNS AND REFOCUS ON THE THINGS THAT MAKE
YOU HAPPY AND GRATEFUL.

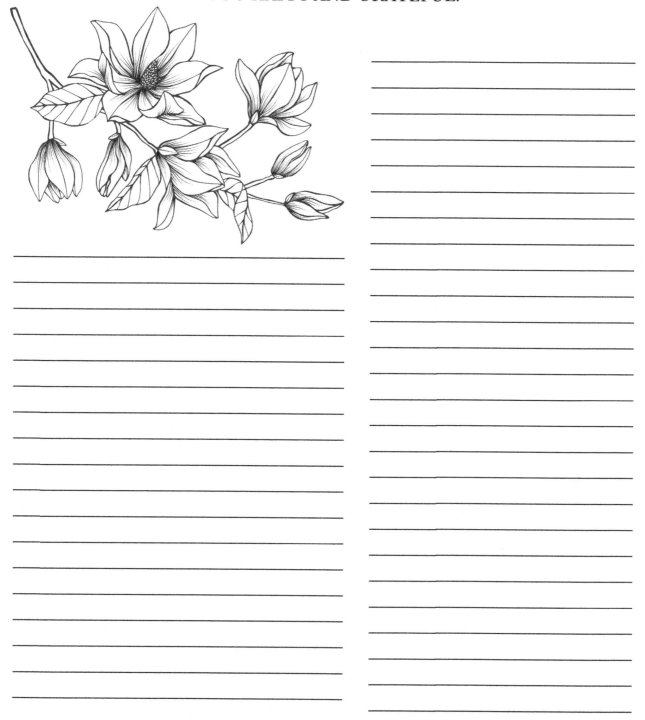

DAILY ENERGY VS MOOD TRACKER

TRACK YOUR DAILY ENERGY AND MOOD, AS WELL AS DETAILS IN THE NOTES SECTION TO SPOT TRIGGERS.

100

75

50

25

0   MONDAY   TUESDAY   WEDNESDAY   THURSDAY   FRIDAY   SATURDAY   SUNDAY

FATIGUE/ENERGY   MOOD/ ANXIETYY

FERTILITY TRACKER

CYCLE DAY	1	2	3	4	5	6	7	8	9	10
DATE										
DAY OF THE WEEK										
INTERCOURSE Y/N										
WAKING TEMP.										
CERVICAL FLUID Y/N										
CERVICAL FLUID KEY FOR TYPES	EGGWHITE LIKE (E) SLIPPERY, STRETCHY		CREAMY (C) OPAQUE, MILKY, LOTION-LIKE		STICKY (S) RUBBERY, CRUMBLES, CEMENT		BLEEDING (B)		Use this key to track your cervical fluid changes below.	
CERVICAL FLUID TYPE										
OVULATION Y/N										
OVULATION PAIN Y/N										
LH SPIKE										
STRESS Y/N										
ILLNESS Y/N										
SORE BREASTS Y/N										
CRAMPING										
MOOD TYPE KEY	HORMONAL, (E) MOOD SWINGS, EMOTIONAL		CALM, (C) NEUTRAL, DAY-TO-DAY		ANXIOUS, (S) DEPRESSED, STRESSED.		HAPPY, (H) ENERGETIC.		Use this key to track your mood changes below.	
MOOD										
BLOATING										

MEDICATION & SUPPLEMENT TRACKING & DOSE

CYCLE DAY	1	2	3	4	5	6	7	8	9	10
MEDICATION NAME EXAMPLE	DOSE	N/A								

FERTILITY TRACKER

CYCLE DAY	11	12	13	14	15	16	17	18	19	20
DATE										
DAY OF THE WEEK										
INTERCOURSE Y/N										
WAKING TEMP.										
CERVICAL FLUID Y/N										
CERVICAL FLUID KEY FOR TYPES	EGGWHITE LIKE Ⓔ SLIPPERY, STRETCHY		CREAMY Ⓒ OPAQUE, MILKY, LOTION-LIKE		STICKY Ⓢ RUBBERY, CRUMBLES, CEMENT		BLEEDING Ⓑ		Use this key to track your cervical fluid changes below.	
CERVICAL FLUID TYPE										
OVULATION Y/N										
OVULATION PAIN Y/N										
LH SPIKE										
STRESS Y/N										
ILLNESS Y/N										
SORE BREASTS Y/N										
CRAMPING										
MOOD TYPE KEY	HORMONAL, Ⓔ MOOD SWINGS, EMOTIONAL		CALM, Ⓒ NEUTRAL, DAY-TO-DAY		ANXIOUS, Ⓢ DEPRESSED, STRESSED.		HAPPY, Ⓗ ENERGETIC.		Use this key to track your mood changes below.	
MOOD										
BLOATING										

MEDICATION & SUPPLEMENT TRACKING & DOSE

CYCLE DAY	11	12	13	14	15	16	17	18	19	20
MEDICATION NAME EXAMPLE	DOSE	N/A								

FERTILITY TRACKER

CYCLE DAY	21	22	23	24	25	26	27	28	29	30
DATE										
DAY OF THE WEEK										
INTERCOURSE Y/N										
WAKING TEMP.										
CERVICAL FLUID Y/N										
CERVICAL FLUID KEY FOR TYPES	EGGWHITE LIKE, SLIPPERY, STRETCHY (E)	CREAMY OPAQUE, MILKY, LOTION-LIKE (C)	STICKY RUBBERY, CRUMBLES, CEMENT (S)		BLEEDING (B)				Use this key to track your cervical fluid changes below.	
CERVICAL FLUID TYPE										
OVULATION Y/N										
OVULATION PAIN Y/N										
LH SPIKE										
STRESS Y/N										
ILLNESS Y/N										
SORE BREASTS Y/N										
CRAMPING										
MOOD TYPE KEY	HORMONAL, MOOD SWINGS, EMOTIONAL (E)	CALM, NEUTRAL, DAY-TO-DAY (C)	ANXIOUS, DEPRESSED, STRESSED. (S)		HAPPY, ENERGETIC. (H)				Use this key to track your mood changes below.	
MOOD										
BLOATING										

MEDICATION & SUPPLEMENT TRACKING & DOSE

CYCLE DAY	21	22	23	24	25	26	27	28	29	30
MEDICATION NAME EXAMPLE	DOSE	N/A								

FERTILITY TRACKER

CYCLE DAY	31	32	33	34	35	36	37	38	39	40
DATE										
DAY OF THE WEEK										
INTERCOURSE Y/N										
WAKING TEMP.										
CERVICAL FLUID Y/N										
CERVICAL FLUID KEY FOR TYPES	EGGWHITE LIKE, SLIPPERY, STRETCHY (E)	CREAMY OPAQUE, MILKY, LOTION-LIKE (C)	STICKY RUBBERY, CRUMBLES, CEMENT (S)		BLEEDING (B)		Use this key to track your cervical fluid changes below.			
CERVICAL FLUID TYPE										
OVULATION Y/N										
OVULATION PAIN Y/N										
LH SPIKE										
STRESS Y/N										
ILLNESS Y/N										
SORE BREASTS Y/N										
CRAMPING										
MOOD TYPE KEY	HORMONAL, MOOD SWINGS, EMOTIONAL (E)	CALM, NEUTRAL, DAY-TO-DAY (C)	ANXIOUS, DEPRESSED, STRESSED. (S)		HAPPY, ENERGETIC. (H)		Use this key to track your mood changes below.			
MOOD										
BLOATING										

MEDICATION & SUPPLEMENT TRACKING & DOSE

CYCLE DAY	31	32	33	34	35	36	37	38	39	40
MEDICATION NAME EXAMPLE	DOSE	N/A								

MEDICATION LOG WEEK_____ CYCLE _____ DATE _____

CYCLE DAY / MEDICATION	1	2	3	4	5	6	7	8	9	10
MEDICATION NAME EXAMPLE	DOSE TIMESTAMP									

CYCLE DAY / MEDICATION	11	12	13	14	15	16	17	18	19	20

CYCLE DAY MEDICATION	21	22	23	24	25	26	27	28	29	30
MEDICATION NAME EXAMPLE	DOSE TIMESTAMP									

CYCLE DAY MEDICATION	31	32	33	34	35	36	37	38	39	40

RESULTS, HORMONE AND SYMPTOM LOG   WEEK_____ CYCLE _____ DATE _____

CYCLE DAY / RESULTS & SYMPTOMS	1	2	3	4	5	6	7	8	9	10
DATE										
BASAL TEMP										
LH										
PROGESTERONE										
OESTROGEN										
ENDOTHICKNESS										
FOLLICLES RIGHT # & SIZE										
FOLLICLES LEFT # & SIZE										
FILL IN YOUR OWN										

CYCLE DAY / RESULTS & SYMPTOMS	11	12	13	14	15	16	17	18	19	20
DATE										
BASAL TEMP										
LH										
PROGESTERONE										
OESTROGEN										
ENDOTHICKNESS										
FOLLICLES RIGHT # & SIZE										
FOLLICLES LEFT # & SIZE										
FILL IN YOUR OWN										

RESULTS, HORMONE AND SYMPTOM LOG   WEEK_____ CYCLE _____ DATE _____

CYCLE DAY / RESULTS & SYMPTOMS	21	22	23	24	25	26	27	28	29	30
DATE										
BASAL TEMP										
LH										
PROGESTERONE										
OESTROGEN										
ENDOTHICKNESS										
FOLLICLES RIGHT # & SIZE										
FOLLICLES LEFT # & SIZE										
FILL IN YOUR OWN										

CYCLE DAY / RESULTS & SYMPTOMS	31	32	33	34	35	36	37	38	39	40
DATE										
BASAL TEMP										
LH										
PROGESTERONE										
OESTROGEN										
ENDOTHICKNESS										
FOLLICLES RIGHT # & SIZE										
FOLLICLES LEFT # & SIZE										
FILL IN YOUR OWN										

SYMPTOM TRACKER

DATE	TIME	DURATION	DESCRIPTION
DATE	TIME	DURATION	DESCRIPTION

DOCTORS APPOINTMENTS TIME SHEET

DATE	TIME	DOCTOR & LOCATION	REASON & NOTES

EMERGENCY & DOCTORS CONTACTS

_____

_____

_____

_____

_____

_____

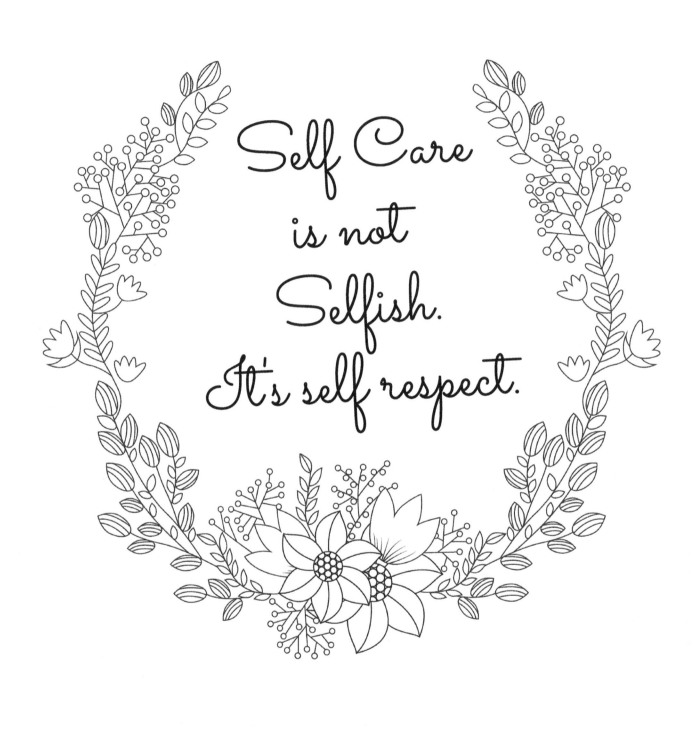

Self Care
is not
Selfish.
It's self respect.

MONTH:

1 2 3 4 5 6 7 8 9 10

11 12 13 14 15 16 17 18 19

20 21 22 23 24 25 26 27 28

29 30 31

MONTH:

1 2 3 4 5 6 7 8 9 10

11 12 13 14 15 16 17 18 19

20 21 22 23 24 25 26 27 28

29 30 31

MONTH:

1 2 3 4 5 6 7 8 9 10

11 12 13 14 15 16 17 18 19

20 21 22 23 24 25 26 27 28

29 30 31

WHEN IS IT IMPORTANT TO FEEL GRATITUDE?

ANSWER THESE QUESTIONS TO BREAK OUT OF NEGATIVE THOUGHT PATTERNS AND REFOCUS ON THE THINGS THAT MAKE YOU HAPPY AND GRATEFUL.

_____

_____

_____

_____

_____

_____

_____

_____

_____

_____

_____

_____

_____

_____

_____

_____

_____

_____

_____

_____

_____

DAILY ENERGY VS MOOD TRACKER

TRACK YOUR DAILY ENERGY AND MOOD, AS WELL AS DETAILS IN THE NOTES SECTION TO SPOT TRIGGERS.

| | 100 | | | | | | | 😄 |

| | 75 | | | | | | | 😌 |

| | 50 | | | | | | | 😐 |

| | 25 | | | | | | | ☹️ |

| | 0 | MONDAY | TUESDAY | WEDNESDAY | THURSDAY | FRIDAY | SATURDAY | SUNDAY | 😫 |

FATIGUE/ENERGY   MOOD/ ANXIETYY

_____

_____

_____

_____

_____

_____

_____

_____

_____

_____

_____

_____

_____

_____

_____

_____

_____

_____

_____

_____

_____

_____

FERTILITY TRACKER

CYCLE DAY	1	2	3	4	5	6	7	8	9	10
DATE										
DAY OF THE WEEK										
INTERCOURSE Y/N										
WAKING TEMP.										
CERVICAL FLUID Y/N										
CERVICAL FLUID KEY FOR TYPES	EGGWHITE LIKE (E) SLIPPERY, STRETCHY		CREAMY (C) OPAQUE, MILKY, LOTION-LIKE		STICKY (S) RUBBERY, CRUMBLES, CEMENT		BLEEDING (B)		Use this key to track your cervical fluid changes below.	
CERVICAL FLUID TYPE										
OVULATION Y/N										
OVULATION PAIN Y/N										
LH SPIKE										
STRESS Y/N										
ILLNESS Y/N										
SORE BREASTS Y/N										
CRAMPING										
MOOD TYPE KEY	HORMONAL, (E) MOOD SWINGS, EMOTIONAL		CALM, (C) NEUTRAL, DAY-TO-DAY		ANXIOUS, (S) DEPRESSED, STRESSED.		HAPPY, (H) ENERGETIC.		Use this key to track your mood changes below.	
MOOD										
BLOATING										

MEDICATION & SUPPLEMENT TRACKING & DOSE

CYCLE DAY	1	2	3	4	5	6	7	8	9	10
MEDICATION NAME EXAMPLE	DOSE	N/A								

FERTILITY TRACKER

CYCLE DAY	11	12	13	14	15	16	17	18	19	20
DATE										
DAY OF THE WEEK										
INTERCOURSE Y/N										
WAKING TEMP.										
CERVICAL FLUID Y/N										
CERVICAL FLUID KEY FOR TYPES	EGGWHITE LIKE SLIPPERY, STRETCHY (E)		CREAMY OPAQUE, MILKY, LOTION-LIKE (C)		STICKY RUBBERY, CRUMBLES, CEMENT (S)		BLEEDING (B)		Use this key to track your cervical fluid changes below.	
CERVICAL FLUID TYPE										
OVULATION Y/N										
OVULATION PAIN Y/N										
LH SPIKE										
STRESS Y/N										
ILLNESS Y/N										
SORE BREASTS Y/N										
CRAMPING										
MOOD TYPE KEY	HORMONAL, MOOD SWINGS, EMOTIONAL (E)		CALM, NEUTRAL, DAY-TO-DAY (C)		ANXIOUS, DEPRESSED, STRESSED. (S)		HAPPY, ENERGETIC. (H)		Use this key to track your mood changes below.	
MOOD										
BLOATING										

MEDICATION & SUPPLEMENT TRACKING & DOSE

CYCLE DAY	11	12	13	14	15	16	17	18	19	20
MEDICATION NAME EXAMPLE	DOSE	N/A								

FERTILITY TRACKER

CYCLE DAY	21	22	23	24	25	26	27	28	29	30
DATE										
DAY OF THE WEEK										
INTERCOURSE Y/N										
WAKING TEMP.										
CERVICAL FLUID Y/N										
CERVICAL FLUID KEY FOR TYPES	EGGWHITE LIKE (E) SLIPPERY, STRETCHY		CREAMY (C) OPAQUE, MILKY, LOTION-LIKE		STICKY (S) RUBBERY, CRUMBLES, CEMENT		BLEEDING (B)		Use this key to track your cervical fluid changes below.	
CERVICAL FLUID TYPE										
OVULATION Y/N										
OVULATION PAIN Y/N										
LH SPIKE										
STRESS Y/N										
ILLNESS Y/N										
SORE BREASTS Y/N										
CRAMPING										
MOOD TYPE KEY	HORMONAL, (E) MOOD SWINGS, EMOTIONAL		CALM, (C) NEUTRAL, DAY-TO-DAY		ANXIOUS, (S) DEPRESSED, STRESSED.		HAPPY, (H) ENERGETIC.		Use this key to track your mood changes below.	
MOOD										
BLOATING										

MEDICATION & SUPPLEMENT TRACKING & DOSE

CYCLE DAY	21	22	23	24	25	26	27	28	29	30
MEDICATION NAME EXAMPLE	DOSE	N/A								

FERTILITY TRACKER

CYCLE DAY	31	32	33	34	35	36	37	38	39	40
DATE										
DAY OF THE WEEK										
INTERCOURSE Y/N										
WAKING TEMP.										
CERVICAL FLUID Y/N										
CERVICAL FLUID KEY FOR TYPES	EGGWHITE LIKE SLIPPERY, STRETCHY (E)		CREAMY OPAQUE, MILKY, LOTION-LIKE (C)		STICKY RUBBERY, CRUMBLES, CEMENT (S)		BLEEDING (B)		Use this key to track your cervical fluid changes below.	
CERVICAL FLUID TYPE										
OVULATION Y/N										
OVULATION PAIN Y/N										
LH SPIKE										
STRESS Y/N										
ILLNESS Y/N										
SORE BREASTS Y/N										
CRAMPING										
MOOD TYPE KEY	HORMONAL, MOOD SWINGS, EMOTIONAL (E)		CALM, NEUTRAL, DAY-TO-DAY (C)		ANXIOUS, DEPRESSED, STRESSED. (S)		HAPPY, ENERGETIC. (H)		Use this key to track your mood changes below.	
MOOD										
BLOATING										

MEDICATION & SUPPLEMENT TRACKING & DOSE

CYCLE DAY	31	32	33	34	35	36	37	38	39	40
MEDICATION NAME EXAMPLE	DOSE	N/A								

MEDICATION LOG   WEEK_____ CYCLE _____ DATE _____

CYCLE DAY / MEDICATION	1	2	3	4	5	6	7	8	9	10
MEDICATION NAME EXAMPLE	DOSE TIMESTAMP									

CYCLE DAY / MEDICATION	11	12	13	14	15	16	17	18	19	20

MEDICATION LOG		WEEK_____		CYCLE _____		DATE _____			
CYCLE DAY MEDICATION	21	22	23	24	25	26	27	28	29	30
MEDICATION NAME EXAMPLE	DOSE TIMESTAMP									

CYCLE DAY MEDICATION	31	32	33	34	35	36	37	38	39	40

RESULTS, HORMONE AND SYMPTOM LOG   WEEK_____ CYCLE _____ DATE _____

CYCLE DAY / RESULTS & SYMPTOMS	1	2	3	4	5	6	7	8	9	10
DATE										
BASAL TEMP										
LH										
PROGESTERONE										
OESTROGEN										
ENDOTHICKNESS										
FOLLICLES RIGHT # & SIZE										
FOLLICLES LEFT # & SIZE										
FILL IN YOUR OWN										

CYCLE DAY / RESULTS & SYMPTOMS	11	12	13	14	15	16	17	18	19	20
DATE										
BASAL TEMP										
LH										
PROGESTERONE										
OESTROGEN										
ENDOTHICKNESS										
FOLLICLES RIGHT # & SIZE										
FOLLICLES LEFT # & SIZE										
FILL IN YOUR OWN										

RESULTS, HORMONE AND SYMPTOM LOG   WEEK_____ CYCLE _____ DATE _____

CYCLE DAY RESULTS & SYMPTOMS	21	22	23	24	25	26	27	28	29	30
DATE										
BASAL TEMP										
LH										
PROGESTERONE										
OESTROGEN										
ENDOTHICKNESS										
FOLLICLES RIGHT # & SIZE										
FOLLICLES LEFT # & SIZE										
FILL IN YOUR OWN										

CYCLE DAY RESULTS & SYMPTOMS	31	32	33	34	35	36	37	38	39	40
DATE										
BASAL TEMP										
LH										
PROGESTERONE										
OESTROGEN										
ENDOTHICKNESS										
FOLLICLES RIGHT # & SIZE										
FOLLICLES LEFT # & SIZE										
FILL IN YOUR OWN										

SYMPTOM TRACKER

DATE	TIME	DURATION	DESCRIPTION

DOCTORS APPOINTMENTS TIME SHEET

DATE	TIME	DOCTOR & LOCATION	REASON & NOTES

EMERGENCY & DOCTORS CONTACTS

MONTH:

1 2 3 4 5 6 7 8 9 10

11 12 13 14 15 16 17 18 19

20 21 22 23 24 25 26 27 28

29 30 31

MONTH:

1 2 3 4 5 6 7 8 9 10

11 12 13 14 15 16 17 18 19

20 21 22 23 24 25 26 27 28

29 30 31

MONTH:

1 2 3 4 5 6 7 8 9 10

11 12 13 14 15 16 17 18 19

20 21 22 23 24 25 26 27 28

29 30 31

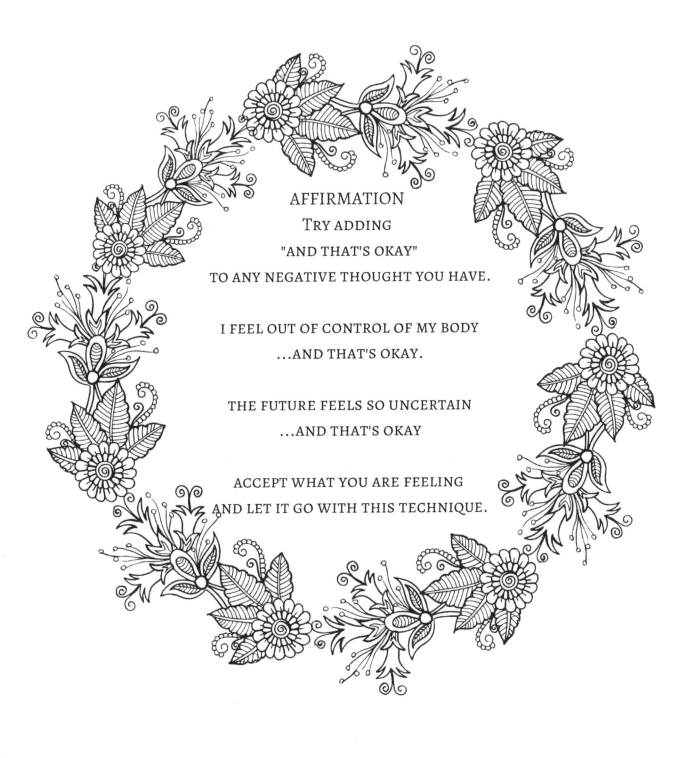

AFFIRMATION
TRY ADDING
"AND THAT'S OKAY"
TO ANY NEGATIVE THOUGHT YOU HAVE.

I FEEL OUT OF CONTROL OF MY BODY
...AND THAT'S OKAY.

THE FUTURE FEELS SO UNCERTAIN
...AND THAT'S OKAY

ACCEPT WHAT YOU ARE FEELING
AND LET IT GO WITH THIS TECHNIQUE.

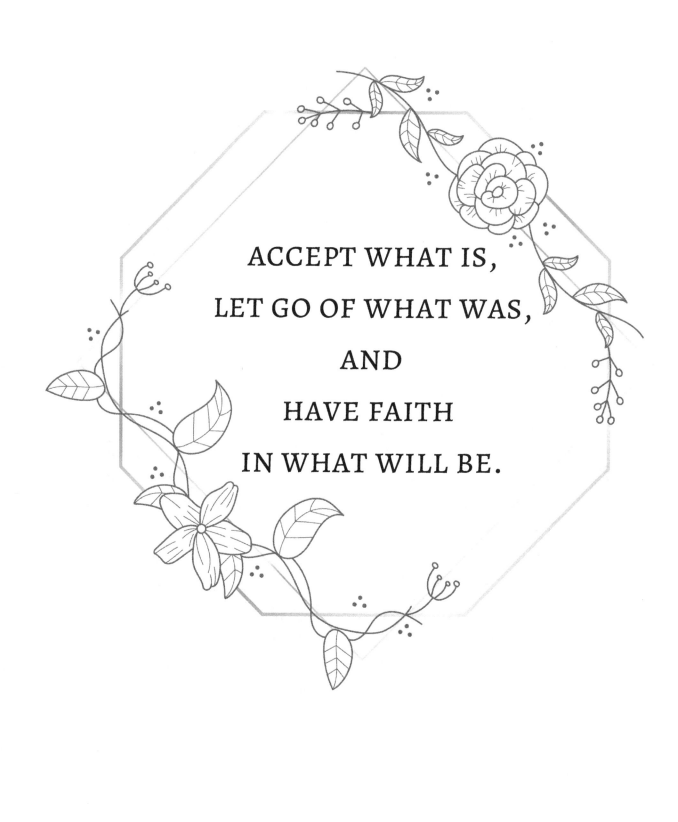

ACCEPT WHAT IS,

LET GO OF WHAT WAS,

AND

HAVE FAITH

IN WHAT WILL BE.

DAILY ENERGY VS MOOD TRACKER

TRACK YOUR DAILY ENERGY AND MOOD, AS WELL AS DETAILS IN THE NOTES SECTION TO SPOT TRIGGERS.

100	
75	
50	
25	
0	MONDAY TUESDAY WEDNESDAY THURSDAY FRIDAY SATURDAY SUNDAY

FATIGUE/ENERGY

MOOD/ ANXIETYY

FERTILITY TRACKER

CYCLE DAY	1	2	3	4	5	6	7	8	9	10
DATE										
DAY OF THE WEEK										
INTERCOURSE Y/N										
WAKING TEMP.										
CERVICAL FLUID Y/N										
CERVICAL FLUID KEY FOR TYPES	EGGWHITE LIKE (E) SLIPPERY, STRETCHY		CREAMY (C) OPAQUE, MILKY, LOTION-LIKE		STICKY (S) RUBBERY, CRUMBLES, CEMENT		BLEEDING (B)		Use this key to track your cervical fluid changes below.	
CERVICAL FLUID TYPE										
OVULATION Y/N										
OVULATION PAIN Y/N										
LH SPIKE										
STRESS Y/N										
ILLNESS Y/N										
SORE BREASTS Y/N										
CRAMPING										
MOOD TYPE KEY	HORMONAL, (E) MOOD SWINGS, EMOTIONAL		CALM, (C) NEUTRAL, DAY-TO-DAY		ANXIOUS, (S) DEPRESSED, STRESSED.		HAPPY, (H) ENERGETIC.		Use this key to track your mood changes below.	
MOOD										
BLOATING										

MEDICATION & SUPPLEMENT TRACKING & DOSE

CYCLE DAY	1	2	3	4	5	6	7	8	9	10
MEDICATION NAME EXAMPLE	DOSE	N/A								

FERTILITY TRACKER

CYCLE DAY	11	12	13	14	15	16	17	18	19	20
DATE										
DAY OF THE WEEK										
INTERCOURSE Y/N										
WAKING TEMP.										
CERVICAL FLUID Y/N										
CERVICAL FLUID KEY FOR TYPES	EGGWHITE LIKE SLIPPERY, STRETCHY (E)	CREAMY OPAQUE, MILKY, LOTION-LIKE (C)	STICKY RUBBERY, CRUMBLES, CEMENT (S)		BLEEDING (B)			Use this key to track your cervical fluid changes below.		
CERVICAL FLUID TYPE										
OVULATION Y/N										
OVULATION PAIN Y/N										
LH SPIKE										
STRESS Y/N										
ILLNESS Y/N										
SORE BREASTS Y/N										
CRAMPING										
MOOD TYPE KEY	HORMONAL, MOOD SWINGS, EMOTIONAL (E)	CALM, NEUTRAL, DAY-TO-DAY (C)	ANXIOUS, DEPRESSED, STRESSED. (S)		HAPPY, ENERGETIC. (H)			Use this key to track your mood changes below.		
MOOD										
BLOATING										

MEDICATION & SUPPLEMENT TRACKING & DOSE

CYCLE DAY	11	12	13	14	15	16	17	18	19	20
MEDICATION NAME EXAMPLE	DOSE	N/A								

FERTILITY TRACKER

CYCLE DAY	21	22	23	24	25	26	27	28	29	30
DATE										
DAY OF THE WEEK										
INTERCOURSE Y/N										
WAKING TEMP.										
CERVICAL FLUID Y/N										
CERVICAL FLUID KEY FOR TYPES	EGGWHITE LIKE (E) SLIPPERY, STRETCHY		CREAMY (C) OPAQUE, MILKY, LOTION-LIKE		STICKY (S) RUBBERY, CRUMBLES, CEMENT		BLEEDING (B)		Use this key to track your cervical fluid changes below.	
CERVICAL FLUID TYPE										
OVULATION Y/N										
OVULATION PAIN Y/N										
LH SPIKE										
STRESS Y/N										
ILLNESS Y/N										
SORE BREASTS Y/N										
CRAMPING										
MOOD TYPE KEY	HORMONAL, (E) MOOD SWINGS, EMOTIONAL		CALM, (C) NEUTRAL, DAY-TO-DAY		ANXIOUS, (S) DEPRESSED, STRESSED.		HAPPY, (H) ENERGETIC.		Use this key to track your mood changes below.	
MOOD										
BLOATING										

MEDICATION & SUPPLEMENT TRACKING & DOSE

CYCLE DAY	21	22	23	24	25	26	27	28	29	30
MEDICATION NAME EXAMPLE	DOSE	N/A								

FERTILITY TRACKER

CYCLE DAY	31	32	33	34	35	36	37	38	39	40
DATE										
DAY OF THE WEEK										
INTERCOURSE Y/N										
WAKING TEMP.										
CERVICAL FLUID Y/N										
CERVICAL FLUID KEY FOR TYPES	EGGWHITE LIKE SLIPPERY, STRETCHY (E)	CREAMY OPAQUE, MILKY, LOTION-LIKE (C)	STICKY RUBBERY, CRUMBLES, CEMENT (S)		BLEEDING (B)		Use this key to track your cervical fluid changes below.			
CERVICAL FLUID TYPE										
OVULATION Y/N										
OVULATION PAIN Y/N										
LH SPIKE										
STRESS Y/N										
ILLNESS Y/N										
SORE BREASTS Y/N										
CRAMPING										
MOOD TYPE KEY	HORMONAL, MOOD SWINGS, EMOTIONAL (E)	CALM, NEUTRAL, DAY-TO-DAY (C)	ANXIOUS, DEPRESSED, STRESSED. (S)		HAPPY, ENERGETIC. (H)		Use this key to track your mood changes below.			
MOOD										
BLOATING										

MEDICATION & SUPPLEMENT TRACKING & DOSE

CYCLE DAY	31	32	33	34	35	36	37	38	39	40
MEDICATION NAME EXAMPLE	DOSE	N/A								

MEDICATION LOG   WEEK_____ CYCLE _____ DATE _____

CYCLE DAY / MEDICATION	1	2	3	4	5	6	7	8	9	10
MEDICATION NAME EXAMPLE	DOSE TIMESTAMP									

CYCLE DAY / MEDICATION	11	12	13	14	15	16	17	18	19	20

MEDICATION LOG   WEEK_____ CYCLE _____ DATE _____

CYCLE DAY / MEDICATION	21	22	23	24	25	26	27	28	29	30
MEDICATION NAME EXAMPLE	DOSE TIMESTAMP									

CYCLE DAY / MEDICATION	31	32	33	34	35	36	37	38	39	40

RESULTS, HORMONE AND SYMPTOM LOG   WEEK_____ CYCLE _____ DATE _____

CYCLE DAY / RESULTS & SYMPTOMS	1	2	3	4	5	6	7	8	9	10
DATE										
BASAL TEMP										
LH										
PROGESTERONE										
OESTROGEN										
ENDOTHICKNESS										
FOLLICLES RIGHT # & SIZE										
FOLLICLES LEFT # & SIZE										
FILL IN YOUR OWN										

CYCLE DAY / RESULTS & SYMPTOMS	11	12	13	14	15	16	17	18	19	20
DATE										
BASAL TEMP										
LH										
PROGESTERONE										
OESTROGEN										
ENDOTHICKNESS										
FOLLICLES RIGHT # & SIZE										
FOLLICLES LEFT # & SIZE										
FILL IN YOUR OWN										

RESULTS, HORMONE AND SYMPTOM LOG   WEEK_____ CYCLE _____ DATE _____

CYCLE DAY / RESULTS & SYMPTOMS	21	22	23	24	25	26	27	28	29	30
DATE										
BASAL TEMP										
LH										
PROGESTERONE										
OESTROGEN										
ENDOTHICKNESS										
FOLLICLES RIGHT # & SIZE										
FOLLICLES LEFT # & SIZE										
FILL IN YOUR OWN										

CYCLE DAY / RESULTS & SYMPTOMS	31	32	33	34	35	36	37	38	39	40
DATE										
BASAL TEMP										
LH										
PROGESTERONE										
OESTROGEN										
ENDOTHICKNESS										
FOLLICLES RIGHT # & SIZE										
FOLLICLES LEFT # & SIZE										
FILL IN YOUR OWN										

SYMPTOM TRACKER

DATE	TIME	DURATION	DESCRIPTION
DATE	TIME	DURATION	DESCRIPTION

DOCTORS APPOINTMENTS TIME SHEET

DATE	TIME	DOCTOR & LOCATION	REASON & NOTES

EMERGENCY & DOCTORS CONTACTS

_____

_____

_____

_____

_____

_____

MONTH:

1 2 3 4 5 6 7 8 9 10

11 12 13 14 15 16 17 18 19

20 21 22 23 24 25 26 27 28

29 30 31

MONTH:

1 2 3 4 5 6 7 8 9 10

11 12 13 14 15 16 17 18 19

20 21 22 23 24 25 26 27 28

29 30 31

MONTH:

1 2 3 4 5 6 7 8 9 10

11 12 13 14 15 16 17 18 19

20 21 22 23 24 25 26 27 28

29 30 31

DAILY ENERGY VS MOOD TRACKER

TRACK YOUR DAILY ENERGY AND MOOD, AS WELL AS DETAILS IN THE NOTES SECTION TO SPOT TRIGGERS.

100

75

50

25

0 MONDAY   TUESDAY   WEDNESDAY   THURSDAY   FRIDAY   SATURDAY   SUNDAY

FATIGUE/ENERGY   MOOD/ ANXIETYY

FERTILITY TRACKER

CYCLE DAY	1	2	3	4	5	6	7	8	9	10
DATE										
DAY OF THE WEEK										
INTERCOURSE Y/N										
WAKING TEMP.										
CERVICAL FLUID Y/N										
CERVICAL FLUID KEY FOR TYPES	EGGWHITE LIKE (E) SLIPPERY, STRETCHY		CREAMY (C) OPAQUE, MILKY, LOTION-LIKE		STICKY (S) RUBBERY, CRUMBLES, CEMENT		BLEEDING (B)		Use this key to track your cervical fluid changes below.	
CERVICAL FLUID TYPE										
OVULATION Y/N										
OVULATION PAIN Y/N										
LH SPIKE										
STRESS Y/N										
ILLNESS Y/N										
SORE BREASTS Y/N										
CRAMPING										
MOOD TYPE KEY	HORMONAL, (E) MOOD SWINGS, EMOTIONAL		CALM, (C) NEUTRAL, DAY-TO-DAY		ANXIOUS, (S) DEPRESSED, STRESSED.		HAPPY, (H) ENERGETIC.		Use this key to track your mood changes below.	
MOOD										
BLOATING										

MEDICATION & SUPPLEMENT TRACKING & DOSE

CYCLE DAY	1	2	3	4	5	6	7	8	9	10
MEDICATION NAME EXAMPLE	DOSE	N/A								

FERTILITY TRACKER

CYCLE DAY	11	12	13	14	15	16	17	18	19	20
DATE										
DAY OF THE WEEK										
INTERCOURSE Y/N										
WAKING TEMP.										
CERVICAL FLUID Y/N										
CERVICAL FLUID KEY FOR TYPES	EGGWHITE LIKE (E) SLIPPERY, STRETCHY		CREAMY (C) OPAQUE, MILKY, LOTION-LIKE		STICKY (S) RUBBERY, CRUMBLES, CEMENT		BLEEDING (B)		Use this key to track your cervical fluid changes below.	
CERVICAL FLUID TYPE										
OVULATION Y/N										
OVULATION PAIN Y/N										
LH SPIKE										
STRESS Y/N										
ILLNESS Y/N										
SORE BREASTS Y/N										
CRAMPING										
MOOD TYPE KEY	HORMONAL, (E) MOOD SWINGS, EMOTIONAL		CALM, (C) NEUTRAL, DAY-TO-DAY		ANXIOUS, (S) DEPRESSED, STRESSED.		HAPPY, (H) ENERGETIC.		Use this key to track your mood changes below.	
MOOD										
BLOATING										

MEDICATION & SUPPLEMENT TRACKING & DOSE

CYCLE DAY	11	12	13	14	15	16	17	18	19	20
MEDICATION NAME EXAMPLE	DOSE	N/A								

FERTILITY TRACKER

CYCLE DAY	21	22	23	24	25	26	27	28	29	30
DATE										
DAY OF THE WEEK										
INTERCOURSE Y/N										
WAKING TEMP.										
CERVICAL FLUID Y/N										
CERVICAL FLUID KEY FOR TYPES	EGGWHITE LIKE (E) SLIPPERY, STRETCHY		CREAMY (C) OPAQUE, MILKY, LOTION-LIKE		STICKY (S) RUBBERY, CRUMBLES, CEMENT		BLEEDING (B)		Use this key to track your cervical fluid changes below.	
CERVICAL FLUID TYPE										
OVULATION Y/N										
OVULATION PAIN Y/N										
LH SPIKE										
STRESS Y/N										
ILLNESS Y/N										
SORE BREASTS Y/N										
CRAMPING										
MOOD TYPE KEY	HORMONAL, (E) MOOD SWINGS, EMOTIONAL		CALM, (C) NEUTRAL, DAY-TO-DAY		ANXIOUS, (S) DEPRESSED, STRESSED.		HAPPY, (H) ENERGETIC.		Use this key to track your mood changes below.	
MOOD										
BLOATING										

MEDICATION & SUPPLEMENT TRACKING & DOSE

CYCLE DAY	21	22	23	24	25	26	27	28	29	30
MEDICATION NAME EXAMPLE	DOSE	N/A								

FERTILITY TRACKER

CYCLE DAY	31	32	33	34	35	36	37	38	39	40
DATE										
DAY OF THE WEEK										
INTERCOURSE Y/N										
WAKING TEMP.										
CERVICAL FLUID Y/N										
CERVICAL FLUID KEY FOR TYPES	EGGWHITE LIKE SLIPPERY, STRETCHY (E)		CREAMY OPAQUE, MILKY, LOTION-LIKE (C)		STICKY RUBBERY, CRUMBLES, CEMENT (S)		BLEEDING	(B)	Use this key to track your cervical fluid changes below.	
CERVICAL FLUID TYPE										
OVULATION Y/N										
OVULATION PAIN Y/N										
LH SPIKE										
STRESS Y/N										
ILLNESS Y/N										
SORE BREASTS Y/N										
CRAMPING										
MOOD TYPE KEY	HORMONAL, MOOD SWINGS, EMOTIONAL (E)		CALM, NEUTRAL, DAY-TO-DAY (C)		ANXIOUS, DEPRESSED, STRESSED. (S)		HAPPY, ENERGETIC. (H)		Use this key to track your mood changes below.	
MOOD										
BLOATING										

MEDICATION & SUPPLEMENT TRACKING & DOSE

CYCLE DAY	31	32	33	34	35	36	37	38	39	40
MEDICATION NAME EXAMPLE	DOSE	N/A								

MEDICATION LOG   WEEK_____ CYCLE _____ DATE _____

CYCLE DAY / MEDICATION	1	2	3	4	5	6	7	8	9	10
MEDICATION NAME EXAMPLE	DOSE TIMESTAMP									

CYCLE DAY / MEDICATION	11	12	13	14	15	16	17	18	19	20

SYMPTOM TRACKER

DATE	TIME	DURATION	DESCRIPTION

DOCTORS APPOINTMENTS TIME SHEET

DATE	TIME	DOCTOR & LOCATION	REASON & NOTES

EMERGENCY & DOCTORS CONTACTS

_____

_____

_____

_____

_____

_____

_____

TWO WEEK WAIT

WHAT I DID TODAY

MONDAY
_____
_____

TUESDAY
_____
_____

WEDNESDAY
_____
_____

THURSDAY
_____
_____

FRIDAY
_____
_____

SATURDAY
_____
_____

SUNDAY
_____
_____

TODAY I FELT...

MONDAY
_____
_____

TUESDAY
_____
_____

WEDNESDAY
_____
_____

THURSDAY
_____
_____

FRIDAY
_____
_____

SATURDAY
_____
_____

SUNDAY
_____
_____

TWO WEEK WAIT

WHAT I DID TODAY

MONDAY

_____

_____

TUESDAY

_____

_____

WEDNESDAY

_____

_____

THURSDAY

_____

_____

FRIDAY

_____

_____

SATURDAY

_____

_____

SUNDAY

_____

_____

TODAY I FELT...

MONDAY

_____

_____

TUESDAY

_____

_____

WEDNESDAY

_____

_____

THURSDAY

_____

_____

FRIDAY

_____

_____

SATURDAY

_____

_____

SUNDAY

_____

_____

MONTH:

1 2 3 4 5 6 7 8 9 10

11 12 13 14 15 16 17 18 19

20 21 22 23 24 25 26 27 28

29 30 31

MONTH:

1 2 3 4 5 6 7 8 9 10

11 12 13 14 15 16 17 18 19

20 21 22 23 24 25 26 27 28

29 30 31

MEDICATION LOG   WEEK_____ CYCLE _____ DATE _____

CYCLE DAY / MEDICATION	21	22	23	24	25	26	27	28	29	30
MEDICATION NAME EXAMPLE	DOSE TIMESTAMP									

CYCLE DAY / MEDICATION	31	32	33	34	35	36	37	38	39	40

RESULTS, HORMONE AND SYMPTOM LOG   WEEK_____ CYCLE _____ DATE _____

CYCLE DAY / RESULTS & SYMPTOMS	1	2	3	4	5	6	7	8	9	10
DATE										
BASAL TEMP										
LH										
PROGESTERONE										
OESTROGEN										
ENDOTHICKNESS										
FOLLICLES RIGHT # & SIZE										
FOLLICLES LEFT # & SIZE										
FILL IN YOUR OWN										

CYCLE DAY / RESULTS & SYMPTOMS	11	12	13	14	15	16	17	18	19	20
DATE										
BASAL TEMP										
LH										
PROGESTERONE										
OESTROGEN										
ENDOTHICKNESS										
FOLLICLES RIGHT # & SIZE										
FOLLICLES LEFT # & SIZE										
FILL IN YOUR OWN										

RESULTS, HORMONE AND SYMPTOM LOG   WEEK_____ CYCLE _____ DATE _____

CYCLE DAY RESULTS & SYMPTOMS	21	22	23	24	25	26	27	28	29	30
DATE										
BASAL TEMP										
LH										
PROGESTERONE										
OESTROGEN										
ENDOTHICKNESS										
FOLLICLES RIGHT # & SIZE										
FOLLICLES LEFT # & SIZE										
FILL IN YOUR OWN										

CYCLE DAY RESULTS & SYMPTOMS	31	32	33	34	35	36	37	38	39	40
DATE										
BASAL TEMP										
LH										
PROGESTERONE										
OESTROGEN										
ENDOTHICKNESS										
FOLLICLES RIGHT # & SIZE										
FOLLICLES LEFT # & SIZE										
FILL IN YOUR OWN										

SYMPTOM TRACKER

DATE	TIME	DURATION	DESCRIPTION
DATE	TIME	DURATION	DESCRIPTION

DOCTORS APPOINTMENTS TIME SHEET

DATE	TIME	DOCTOR & LOCATION	REASON & NOTES

EMERGENCY & DOCTORS CONTACTS

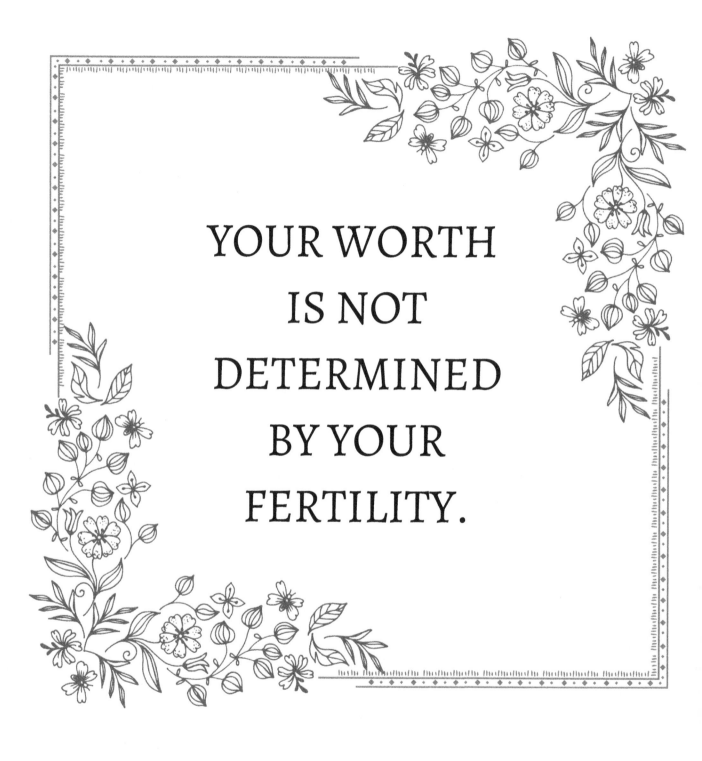

YOUR WORTH
IS NOT
DETERMINED
BY YOUR
FERTILITY.

MONTH:

1 2 3 4 5 6 7 8 9 10

11 12 13 14 15 16 17 18 19

20 21 22 23 24 25 26 27 28

29 30 31

MONTH:

1 2 3 4 5 6 7 8 9 10

11 12 13 14 15 16 17 18 19

20 21 22 23 24 25 26 27 28

29 30 31

43091008R00109